S0-BZU-453

i desperately tried to convince myself that

looks didn't matter. A French egghead said, "Ugliness is superior to beauty because it lasts longer." In other words, screw beauty. Plato said the beauties of the body were nothing compared to the beauties of the soul. In other words, my ugliness was an illusion.

But beauty was too wonderful to be resented or dismissed. I fantasized more about profiles than sex. And I never stopped wanting to be beautiful. Beauty was not goodness, but a visible purity nonetheless. To be made beautiful, free of all flaws, would be a kind of liberation.

And now, a decade later, after the gym and surgery have made me not beautiful, but okay enough to talk face-to-face to beauty queens about perfect skin without making them uneasy, I can begin this trip.

—Ken Siman, *The Beauty Trip*

ALSO AVAILABLE FROM POCKET BOOKS
Pizza Face by Ken Siman

For orders other than by individual consumers, Pocket Books
grants a discount on the purchase of **10 or more copies** of sin-
gle titles for special markets or premium use. For further
details, please write to the Vice-President of Special Markets,
Pocket Books, 1230 Avenue of the Americas, New York, NY
10020

For information on how individual consumers can place
orders, please write to Mail Order Department, Paramount
Publishing, 200 Old Tappan Road, Old Tappan, NJ 07675

the beauty trip • ken siman

POCKET BOOKS

NEW YORK • LONDON • TORONTO • SYDNEY • TOKYO • SINGAPORE

Photograph on page 6:
"Ruth's Skin Care" by Hank O'Neal

The sale of this book without its cover is unauthorized. If you purchased this book without a cover, you should be aware that it was reported to the publisher as "unsold and destroyed." Neither the author nor the publisher has received payment for the sale of this "stripped book."

Publisher and author gratefully acknowledge the *New York Quarterly* for permission to excerpt the Peter Morris poem, "Communist Ice Show."

An *Original* Publication of POCKET BOOKS

 Pocket Books, a division of Simon & Schuster Inc.
1230 Avenue of the Americas, New York, NY 10020

Copyright ©1995 by Ken Siman

All rights reserved, including the right to reproduce this book or portions thereof in any form whatsoever. For information address Pocket Books, 1230 Avenue of the Americas, New York, NY 10020

ISBN: 0-671-89080-8

First Pocket Books trade paperback printing May 1995

10 9 8 7 6 5 4 3 2 1

POCKET and colophon are registered trademarks of Simon & Schuster Inc.

Cover and interior design by Elizabeth Van Itallie

Printed in the U.S.A.

i'm very grateful

to my parents, Eryk Casemiro, Ann Clark, Stephen Gan, Suzanne Gluck,
Dian Griesel, Priscilla Holbrook, James Kaliardos, Richard Pandiscio,
Mary Anne Sacco, David Sedaris, Denise Silvestro, Valerie Steele,
and Elizabeth Van Itallie. I couldn't have written this book without the help
of Shelley Shier and John Siman.

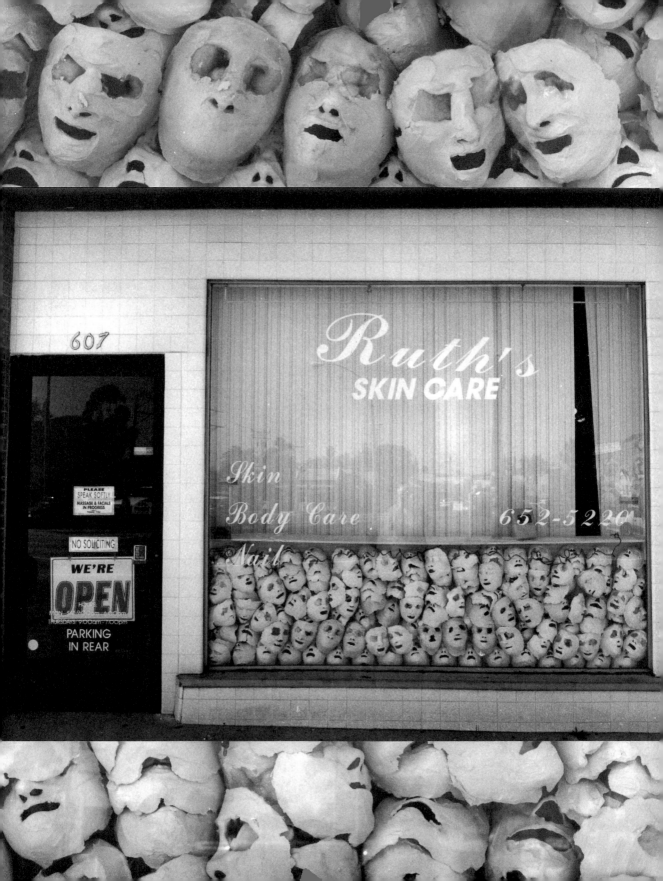

for taro

1

dorothy is an editor at *Playboy*. She and Elly, who is a director at the American Anorexia/Bulimia Association, have come to my apartment. They're getting their makeup done by Billy Beyond before we go to Chippendale's.

Billy's done all the supermodels; he's also a model himself. We've seen him on TV in a wig and makeup, doing runway modeling for Todd Oldham.

Billy is curling Dorothy's eyelashes and sharing his beauty tips with us.

"People look better without plastic surgery unless they've been disfigured," he says. He tells us about a socialite who gets her photo in the "style" sections of newspapers all the time. "She's had so much work done to her face that her makeup, like, slides around. Her skin is so tight it looks plastic."

"You mean the skin's not real?" Dorothy is a little nervous. She once saw a brawl between two tough girls in her high school lavatory. One of the girls had her eye put out by the same beauty utensil Billy's using on her now.

"Keep still, Dorothy," Billy says. "Her skin's real but pulled so tight that it feels weird and looks shiny."

"She does photograph well, though," I say. But evidently some made-for-TV skin looks like plaster in real life. But who, besides Billy, gets that close?

"And can you believe Cher?" he says. "I mean, she used to have this beautiful Cherokee nose. Now she's all pulled and has no nose at all and sells hair-care products while wearing a wig. This is insane!"

Well, no. The beauty trip's risk is not so much insanity but

BELOW: *Cher*
by Roxanne Lowit

RIGHT: *Billy Beyond*
by Roxanne Lowit

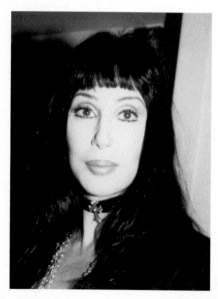

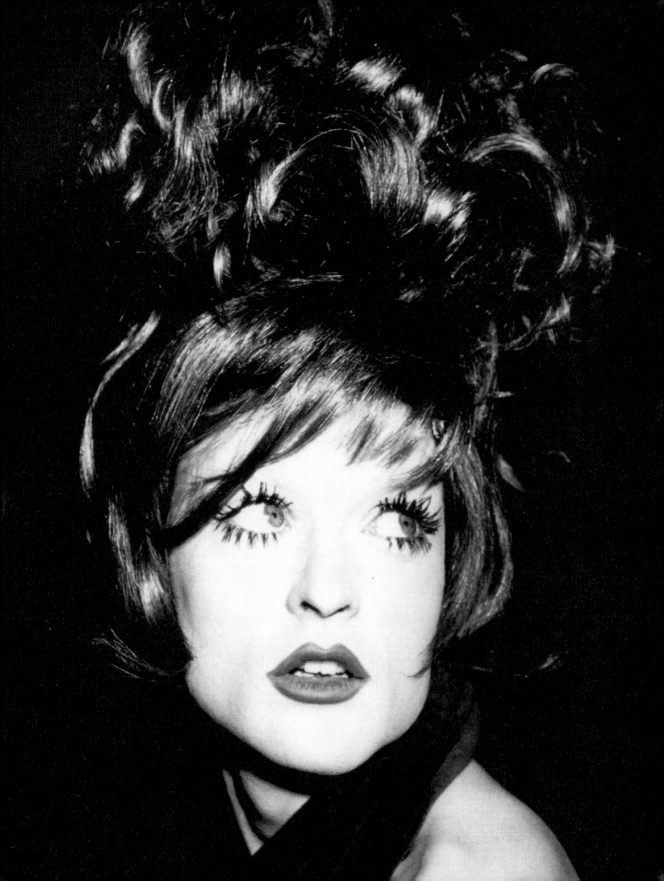

injury. A lot of us preoccupied with beauty have been hurt by it—either by having it severely denied us or by losing it. Anyone who knows the longing that comes with these traumas cannot ignore the promise of a face reinvented by doctors, a body redone by training, or a hair replacement system that doesn't migrate during sex.

That's why I never trash people who try to beautify themselves. I've had some work done myself. I didn't do it to look younger, I'm thirty-one, but because when I was a teenager—and even into my twenties—I had acne so awful that I wore only one contact lens so my face would be blurred when I looked in the mirror. I've always considered mirrors to be the true courtroom of beauty. So when I—my face a combination of blood and benzoyl peroxide—went to this court, I had at least enough instinct for self-preservation to appeal to a half-blind judge.

Being both butt ugly and highly self-conscious of it was not a reflection of my soul, but—at least for a while—of my destiny. By the time I was filling out career questionnaires in college, my fantasy of being a national political figure was shot. If I couldn't cop an invitation to the Mecklenburg County Teenaged Democrats hoedown, how could I stand for U.S. Senate? Josef Stalin, I read, had severe pockmarks, but as a dictator he could have them airbrushed by decree.

Romance, too, was out of the question. With humor and persistence, I could win some dates. But the courtship I wanted, the kind where you make eye contact across campus and fall in love soon after, never happened to me. The eyes connected to the faces I yearned for looked elsewhere.

I desperately tried to convince myself that looks didn't matter. A French egghead said, "Ugliness is superior to beauty because it lasts longer." In other words, fuck beauty. Plato said the beauties of the body were nothing compared to the beauties of the soul. In other words, my ugliness was an illusion.

But beauty was too wonderful to be resented or dismissed. I fantasized more about profiles than sex. And I never stopped wanting to be beautiful. Beauty was not goodness, but a visible purity nonetheless. To be made beautiful, free of all flaws, would be a kind of liberation.

And now, a decade later, after the gym and surgery have made me not beautiful but okay enough to talk face-to-face to beauty queens about perfect skin without making them uneasy, I can begin this trip.

It's now possible to indulge beauty—physical beauty—to an extreme because we are the most leisured culture ever on the face of the earth. Modern technology has made (most) of our bodies irrelevant, except as something to love, loathe, perfect, and decorate.

Also, we—Dorothy, Elly, Billy, and I—come from a generation that never had to confront the kinds of things that would make any lengthy talk of beauty taboo. We never were drafted, we never even protested against a war. Unlike our parents, we never had to struggle or worry through a depression. Unlike our grandparents, we never had to flee tyrants or famines.

Our generation of suburban kids lived out most of our fantasies: money for college was a given. Thanks to the sexual revolution, we were free to choose our lovers and our wardrobes. We all took drugs and if we overdid it, insurance could always pay for rehab. We talked about how we looked and what we wanted to look like, and if we didn't like what we had, we could always change. We started with braces and all wear contacts.

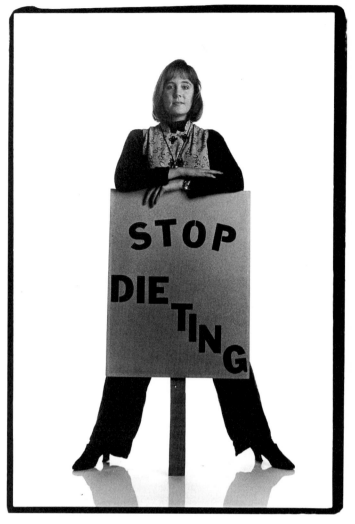

Elly
by Michel Delsol

Elly, who counsels anorexics and bulimics every day, says, "Cher thinks plastic surgery will bring her happiness."

"If it brings her happiness, go for it," says Billy.

Elly is twenty-five. She was pretty enough to be a teenaged shopping mall model. She never had an eating disorder but had friends and a roommate who did. She went to Vassar and founded a peer education group for drug addicts and alcoholics and helped to start one for students with eating disorders. She's been working at the American Anorexia/Bulimia Association (AABA) since she graduated three years ago. Elly's favorite saying is "Don't weigh your self-esteem. It's inside that counts." That's what the poster above her desk says.

It's Elly's job to talk to everyone—the press, students, worried relatives—about eating disorders. This often leads to discussions about diets and beautiful people. So Elly figures it would be "educational" for her to check out Chippendale's.

Elly says if there's only one thing she can get across to women while she's at AABA it's this: Diets don't work. If you want to be lean, exercise and eat healthy, but as a permanent way of life, not as a fad. Never starve yourself or take pills. She's like Carry Nation, except she wants to take an ax to the diet industry instead of a saloon.

"Do you realize how liberated women would be if they stopped obsessing on weight?" Elly says. "Without the ideal inside, you can't reach the ideal outside."

"Wrong," I say. "The world is full of nasty beauties and homely saints. Beauty is the luck of the draw; it's all about what kind of genes you got from your parents."

"What about people who have an outer glow?" says Elly. "Isn't their beauty visible?"

"Their kindness is shining through, their good nature," I say. "But when I talk about beauty, I mean physical beauty."

"If the ideal outside means being so good-looking that photographers stop you on the street and want to take your picture, it has nothing to do with your inside," says Dorothy.

Dorothy should know. Every day at *Playboy,* the photos that men whack off to are in her face. "Most beauties—most models—are very young," Dorothy says. "Some are smart and some are dolts. But they're too young to have a clue about their 'ideal inside.'"

Strangers told Dorothy she was ugly to look at in high school, same as me. When we talk about beauty, we mean the kind of people who can walk in a room and be instantly adored, whether or not they speak. The people who make standing on a long line or in a stalled subway a lot easier, who are stared at, deferred

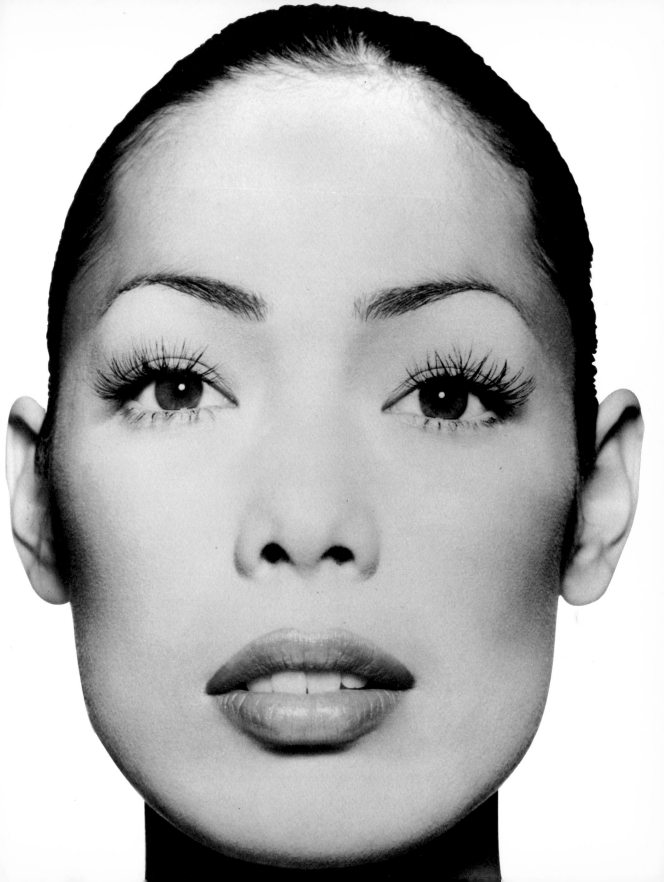

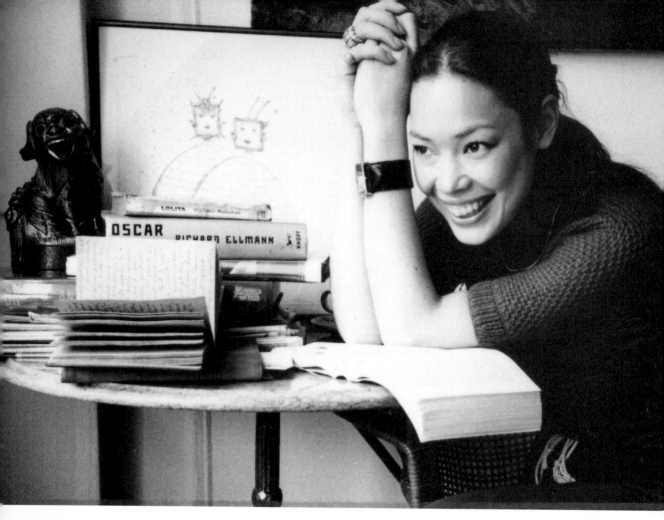

Cecilia
by James Kaliardos

to, and dreamed upon. Dorothy and I don't think beautiful people are media cre-
ations. We started to recognize them in junior high school, before we were staring at magazines. And as we grew up we saw with increasing clarity and
increasing hurt that beauty is very real. The difference between us, though, is
that for Dorothy beauty is more than an aesthetic and more than erotica. Beauty
means power. It's a power she's envied since high school and longed to possess.
Now Dorothy and I are taking this trip together to see the people from the magazines in the flesh, the same people whose photos the rest of the country is mag-
netizing to their refrigerators. "Magazines are the galleries," said the fashion
photographer David LaChapelle. "And the museum is the refrigerator. If someone rips out the photo and puts it on the fridge, that really is something."

Cecilia comes over. She's late because she didn't want to be made up. It
reminds her of her day job. Cecilia is a Click model. There's a huge billboard of

her naked in Times Square—a Benetton ad. Some words cover her erogenous zones. She's done all the magazines—*Vogue*, *Elle*, *Allure*—and *Interview* just named her a "showstopper model."

Cecilia in your living room and Cecilia in the magazines in your living room are two different entities. In the flesh, Cecilia looks like an arty college girl in her peasant skirt and high-top sneakers. "I look much better in photos," she says.

Fashion can be flighty, but there are five traits that models almost always meet. Cecilia has them all. She's tall, five-foot-nine. She has great skin. She's young, twenty-two. She's thin, a size six. And best of all, she photographs beautifully.

Cecilia's half-Chinese. There are more Asian, Hispanic, and black models than ever before—but they are all tall, young, thin, poreless, and look even better when their picture is taken.

Cecilia has brown and yellow hair, but it photographs black. She has freckles on her face, but makeup and lighting erase them when she needs to look older, more glamorous. She can look like a different person in each photo, and that's why she's been able to live in Paris and learn French, travel the world, and have a savings account by twenty-two. The rest of us in the room are older and broke.

It's crazy, Cecilia says, the money she makes. All for standing in front of a camera. "You can't strive or work toward anything," she says. "They're either into you or they're not." If models have more prestige these days, it's because they're the last glamorous women around.

"How can movie stars be magical, mystical, and mythical [when they seem so ordinary]?" Cecilia says. "Garbo and Dietrich wouldn't be able to exist today."

She's right about that. In the age of Dietrich, in the age of Garbo, when Britain still had a colonial empire and America's president accessorized with a cigarette holder and a cape, regular Americans really were curious about the distant world of the rich. Back then the rich were fairy-tale fantasy material. What were the balls like? What were the cafés like? Movie stars, as Gore Vidal has pointed out, let Americans of our parents' generation see life on Olympus.

That kind of aristocracy has evaporated. A Harvard accent and a cigarette holder would be camp today. So would a cinema goddess. "But models can't be demystified," says Cecilia, "because we don't speak."

Some try to demystify beauty by pretending that there's something fair about it, that it somehow makes sense. "Can't we have normal-looking models?" cheerful talk show hosts will scold beauty dictators to applause. "We're *all* beautiful, aren't we, audience?" But beauty—raw physical beauty—the kind that inspires awe, lust, and increased jeans sales, cannot be evenly distributed. In a society where everything is supposed to be within reach, this is painful to face.

So why talk about beauty when it pains many, flusters everybody at one time or another, and often sounds frighteningly shallow in conversation? Maybe I'm dwelling too much on adolescent wounds, still trying to find a perfect prom photo with me in it.

But though I've tried, I've found beauty impossible to ignore. I prefer to face beauty, as intimidating and humbling as that sometimes is, than to force myself to look away. Maybe something so compelling can be an inspiration instead of a whip or a crutch. There must be a way to pursue beauty with grace.

The Chippendale's show starts in fifteen minutes. Billy can't go. He has to work on his new video with Sister Dimension. Their band, Morph, has an album coming out soon.

"Morph as in 'morphine'?"

"No," says Billy. "Morph as in 'metamorphosis.'"

2

the cab's radio is tuned to a top-forty station. When the Madonna song ends, a man from the Center for Nasal Surgery comes on. He says by calling 1-800-545-NOSE you can get a new nose in time for your prom or next important social function. Getting a new nose, he says, is like buying a new car—maybe a sleek European version.

Dorothy has a long nose. She used to try to cover it up with her hands. She went to high school in California in the late seventies and always felt ugly for not having the ideal look of the day, the Farrah Fawcett-Majors look: whirly blond hair, a deep tan, and perky boobs. But Dorothy admits she would have been a gawky teenager in any time.

Dorothy is tall and thin with brown hair as short as a boy's. She used to be afraid to raise her hand in class because it would show how white her skin was. That was before skin cancer was discussed on TV. Now cosmetic surgeons are working on an injection that can turn people tan in an office.

Dorothy got teased for not being a beauty queen, but her parents told her that her nose was beautiful. The aquiline nose was a tradition in her mother's family. She says she came to believe in "the integrity of what I was born with." She likes her nose now, but still gets the uglies, especially when something goes wrong. That's when she thinks "If only I were beautiful...."

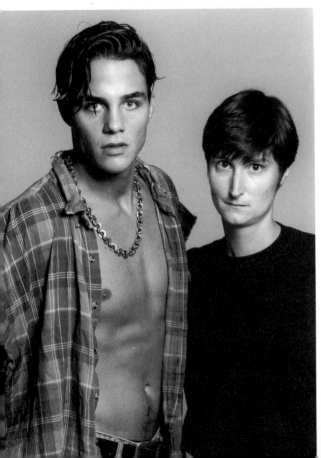

*Mark and Dorothy
by Christopher Makos*

OVERLEAF: *Mark
by Christopher Makos*

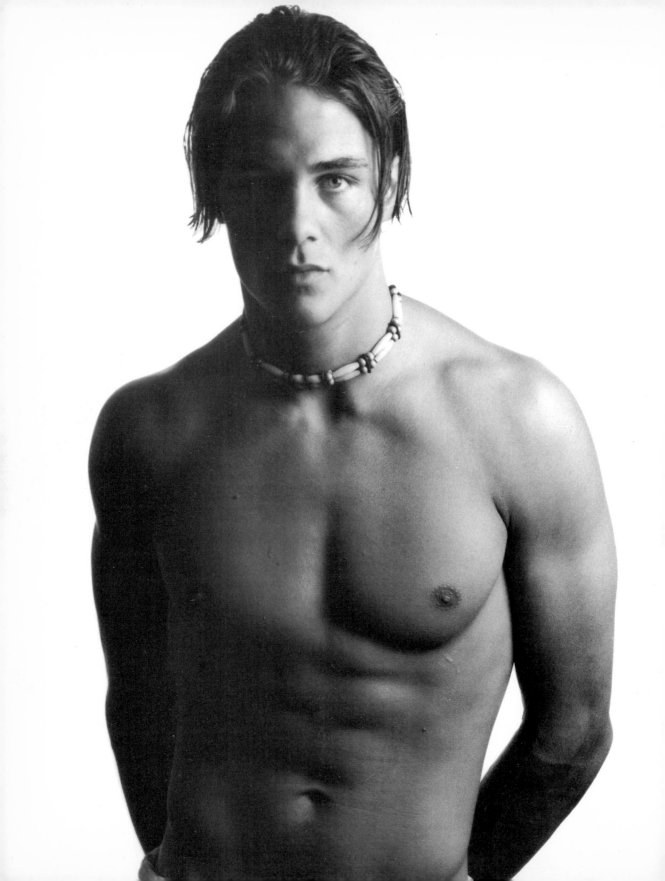

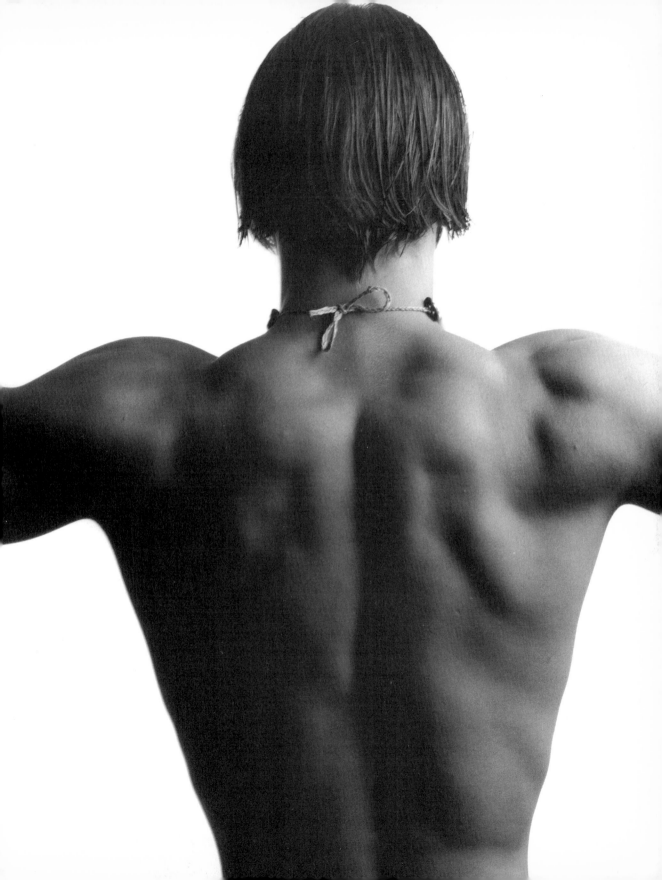

Chippendale's facade looks like the outside of a suburban movie theater: white and windowless. A little bald man tells us that it's twenty dollars to get in, ten dollars extra to sit in the front row. There's a two-drink minimum, and you have to pay for everything now.

Men who aren't bare-chested can't sit with the women. So I have to go above it all, to the "VIP Room" upstairs. There's a glass partition between me and the live action. I'm all alone up here except for two dancers who are getting ready for the show. One of them is doing push-ups.

"Do what you want to do," his friend says. "I'm doing my nails."

The guys at Chippendale's have been apparently flawless since birth and now have perfect gym and grooming routines. No pimples, no cowlicks, nothing close to a love handle. A lot of muscles and expensive haircuts. They all look like clean-cut college boys except for two with neatly groomed shoulder-length hair. Their physiques are no different from those of fifth-century Greek hunks. They could be molded into statues if the women poured plaster of Paris on them instead of dollar bills.

The waiters wear bow ties over shirtless chests and balance cocktails on a tray. They are pretty muscle-boy versions of the extinct *Playboy* bunny.

The faces are so pretty and the hair so well managed that I wonder if most of these guys are gay. But I hear them call each other "dude" a lot more than "girl-friend." My waiter, Mark, is a twenty-one-year-old Ford model. He says most of the dancers are straight, and want to model or act. Mark's girlfriend is a soap opera vixen.

"What's it like having all those women ogle you?"

"It's a trip, man."

"Uh, could you be more specific?"

"It's like bunjee jumping."

"Do gay guys hit on you a lot?"

Gay guys are cool, Mark says, but sometimes they cruise him so intensely that he wears sunglasses and a hat when he walks in the West Village and Chelsea.

It's like a gay bar in here. The icons are the same, but then again there's not the smell of too much cologne musked with cigarette smoke.

This is a striptease with a theme. The guys dance in choreographed tribute to

Dracula and *An Officer and a Gentleman,* but they always end the skits showing everything but their fire engines. They lip-synch and simulate fucking towels at the same time. The best part is when the studs go into the audience to kiss the women who hold up dollar bills. The women, all in their twenties and thirties, are giddy but tame. None are by themselves. They all seem to be in groups that are celebrating birthdays or office promotions. Sometimes they hold a bill behind the head of a friend. There are plenty of Instamatic flashes. Nobody puts a bill in a pair of briefs; the guy pecks a cheek and grabs the buck. When his hands get full, he gives the cash to a less muscular Chippendale who follows a few steps behind with a plastic bag.

Cecilia wants more than a peck, she wants to cop a feel.

She gets up from her seat and steps down to the dance floor, a dollar bill clenched in her mouth. But the dude won't kiss the dollar. He grabs it with his hand instead. Tease. She embraces the guy and gets to feel some ass.

"Watch those hands," the emcee says.

Chippendale's calendars and T-shirts are for sale after the show. Unfortunately, there's not a book or instruction manual on how to achieve Chippendale-like abdominal muscles. I've been going to the gym pretty much every day for the last six years, so my pecs and biceps can compete with theirs, but I've not yet been able to get lines in my stomach. And, like I said, their faces are flawless. Some might call their look "plastic," or "too pumped up," or "too pretty," but I couldn't imagine anyone getting upset if one of these guys showed up as a blind date. That's why it costs five dollars just to get your picture taken with a Chippendale.

Before I found a boyfriend, I used to go to nightclubs and parties with my friend Ricardo. He had a wardrobe that took up most of his studio apartment and was arranged alphabetically by designer: Agnès B. to Yamamoto. To me, that was reason enough to defer always to his fashion and beauty advice. Whenever there was a photographer around, Ricardo told me never to pose with a better-looking guy. "Any flaws you have will be accentuated." Ricardo also said to avoid squinting in the sun, because it causes premature crow's-feet.

"Y'all go ahead and get your picture taken," I say to Cecilia, Dorothy, and Elly. "I'll just watch."

Scores, a strip bar for straight guys, is only a few blocks away, so we walk it. It's packed with upper-management men in suits and loosened ties. Lines of company sedans wait outside. "Funny money" for tipping the dancers can be AmExed onto the corporate expense account.

Cecilia, Dorothy, and Elly are the only women here who are wearing tops. A few girls dance onstage, the rest work the room. One of the girls asks Cecilia to dance. "Don't blame me for asking," she says.

The Knicks are playing the Bulls, and there are as many TV monitors as there are girls. It's Scores' "Best o' Both Worlds" policy. Guys can have one eye on Patrick Ewing and the other on Miss Christie Christina.

The girls' salary requirements are piped in over pop rock: A private dance at your table is twenty dollars. If you want the dance to last longer or have the dancer sit down and make conversation, just keep churning out the twenties. The girl working the table behind us has been with the same guy for a half hour. He has a real boner; it's difficult not to notice, even though he's wearing baggy businessman pants, not 501's. The girl is working hard, dancing, caressing her breasts, always making eye contact. Cecilia thinks the dancer's breasts might be made out of silicone, but she cannot be positive since no feelies are allowed. Silicone feels hard, Cecilia says.

Ginger Miller, whose name we know because it says so on the 8 by 10 glossies she's signing, introduces herself. She's escorted by a man in suit, tie, and Instamatic. For ten dollars, Cecilia gets her picture taken with Ginger. "Gosh, honey, you're cute," she tells Cecilia. "You ought to put on a bathing suit and join us."

Elly is transfixed.

"Dorothy, do you think Elly might be AC/DC?" I ask.

"What?"

"Do you think Elly might be bi?"

"I can't hear you."

So we go to the House of Broiled Fish to talk and have a late dinner. Everybody gets the fish of the day and mashed potatoes. Cecilia stays skinny no matter what on account of her high-metabolism genes and youth.

Elly says she's not bi; she just thought the whole spectacle, not the female bodies themselves, was amazing. "Women had so much power there. Did you see how those women had men in the palm of their hands?"

"They were not in power," says Cecilia. "If they were in real power, they'd be running the place, not men."

"That's true," Elly says. "Women should own these bars."

"It's all Mafia," I say.

Elly and Cecilia say Scores was a lot less smarmy than they expected. The girls looked happy, clear-eyed, and—except for silicone—chemical free. A real top-of-the-line joint. But a scaggy one wouldn't be hard to find. It's economics—the richer the clientele, the more glamorous it looks.

"I don't know if this stuff is healthy," says Cecilia. "If we weren't so hung up on sex and bodies, those places wouldn't exist."

"It's all about youth and beauty," says Dorothy. "As long as there are people who look like Chippendale's guys and Scores' girls, there will be a demand to

Cecilia
courtesy of Saks Fifth
Avenue

see them…. Everything tonight was a visual turn-on. It was a magazine come to life. If anybody had wanted actual sex, there are plenty of places to go."

"But they wouldn't have been able to put it on their expense account," says Elly.

Every day, Elly has to hold the hands of women who hate their bodies, who get on a scale every hour, who won't put on a bikini—even when they're alone—who can't enjoy sex, who are afraid to indulge themselves. "Those women tonight were so free with their bodies. It was so liberating," she says.

And even though Chippendale's was kind of cheesy, she says at least

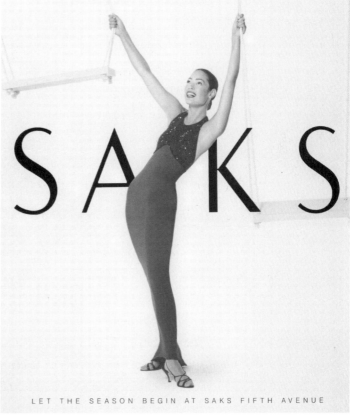

LET THE SEASON BEGIN AT SAKS FIFTH AVENUE

women were allowed to admit they fantasize. A lot of women Elly knows are afraid to masturbate.

"Didn't Madonna help?" I ask. There's that "Like a Virgin" video, where she masturbates in Madison Square Garden.

"Not enough," says Elly.

"Those guys at Chippendale's were hot," says Dorothy. "I mean, I'm a dyke, but I got a rush when I got kissed, even though it was for one second. Can't everybody just admit that it's a rush to be around beautiful young bodies?"

The difference between the two strip joints, says Dorothy, is that the men at Scores had a sense of entitlement. Even the homely guys were at ease with a beautiful woman at their table. The women at Chippendale's were a little nervous about it all.

"Things are changing," says Dorothy. "But men and women will never look at each other's bodies in the same way. Men have always wanted women who are young and beautiful. It's an animal instinct. Youth and beauty are signs of fertility. Of course, women admire attractive guys, but in the end they'd rather have security and status." When those dynamics change, Dorothy says, so will the beauty trip.

"I thought all of this was prostitution at some level," says Cecilia. "But I think modeling is a form of prostitution, as well. They are using their beauty to sell themselves. I use my beauty to sell a product."

Cecilia is hot now, but she knows after tomorrow the phone might never ring, she might never get another modeling job. That's why she's a miser with her money and saves a lot. She's already getting ready for her next career. She just got her B.A. from Columbia and is an editor at *Visionaire,* an art and fashion journal. She wants to edit full-time in the future.

Cecilia wants to know what it's like for Dorothy, a woman editor at *Playboy.*

Dorothy is twenty-nine. She used to be a banker but hated it. She wanted to write and edit and didn't want to wear a suit to work. She was interviewed at *Playboy* by a guy in Levi's and a T-shirt. Her boss is a woman. But at first she felt uglier than ever, having Miss September photos everywhere, until she stopped comparing herself to the models. She doesn't like that type, so why torture herself? Dorothy has photos of beautiful women on her office wall, but it's a

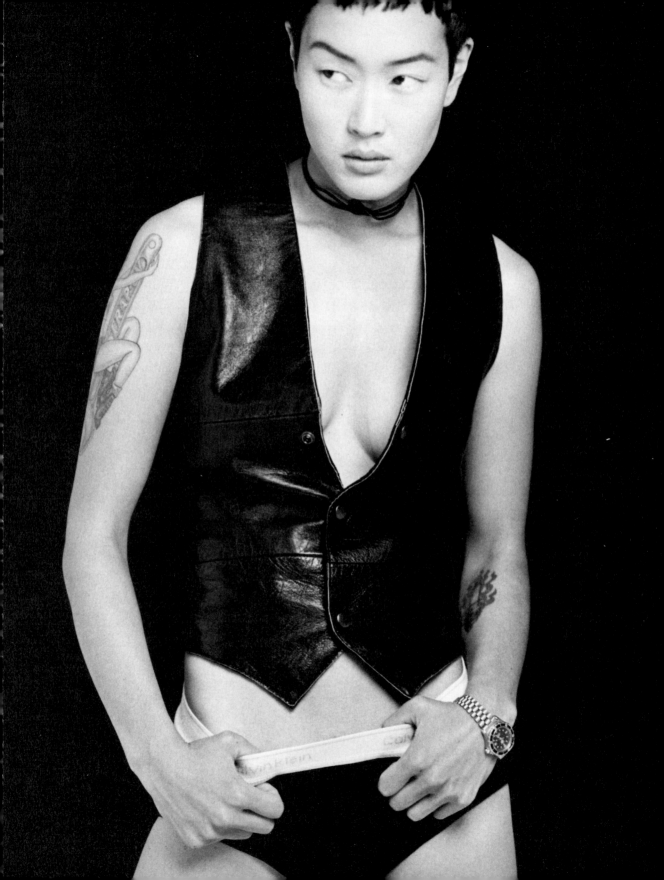

beauty she envies and admires. They are traditional beauties in that they are thin, young, and flawless skinned. But what sets them apart is a boyish edge: short hair, tank tops not tube tops, tattoos instead of big boobs. At first glance, I thought Dorothy's favorite model—Jenny Shimizu—was a beautiful teenaged boy. She was wearing men's briefs.

Dorothy doesn't resent photographs anymore, just social situations. There was a really pretty blond woman just out of college who used to work with Dorothy. They went together to a glitzy *Playboy* party. Dorothy's co-worker "just waltzed in there and had men at her feet." Joe Frazier offered her his phone number. Dorothy didn't want those guys; she didn't want to go down on Joe Frazier. "It's just the acceptance I want, the immediate gratification of having someone look at me right away and smile. I've spent my life working on my personality, getting along with everybody. I know that's more important in the end. But I'll always feel the pain of not being able to go to a party and get that kind of reaction."

"People are jealous of beauty because there's nothing fair about it. You're born with it, or you're not," says Cecilia. Some people are upset with skinny models like Cecilia and the business that pays them. They say most women can never be that tall and a size six. And that's true. "Whenever there's a standard of beauty, a huge majority is not going to be able to attain it," says Cecilia. "Last year it was girls with large breasts, this year it's skinny girls.... If you take this stuff too personally, you'll go crazy."

Cecilia's talking about the standards of the fashion world. But it's the everyday standard that's obsessed Dorothy and me since puberty. It's about possessing the kind of beauty that guarantees strangers will adore you on sight. It's exclusive, of course, but does not require a certain height or weight.

Still, aesthetes like me turn to the fashion world because it allows us to stare shamelessly at amazingly beautiful people without having to worry about being bruised by bouncers or boyfriends, or being served with restraining orders.

3

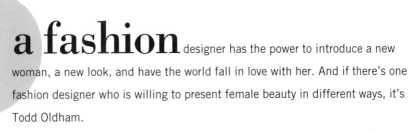

a fashion designer has the power to introduce a new woman, a new look, and have the world fall in love with her. And if there's one fashion designer who is willing to present female beauty in different ways, it's Todd Oldham.

Todd doesn't have portraits of beauty icons in his apartment. He prefers Diane Arbus prints. Todd uses models with crooked noses. One of his favorite models is Billy Beyond in drag.

Todd is thirty-one. He's got an approachable, boyishly cute face. His hair is usually brown, but sometimes it's green or blue.

Todd came to New York from Dallas in 1986 and had his first show two years later. The fashion world wasn't sure what they were supposed to think: models in drag walking down the runway to organ music, the kind that gets played in ice rinks. His designs were out there: a mini-skirt with Mona Lisa on the front and what looks like Marlo Thomas in *That Girl* on the back. But everybody was charmed by Todd. He didn't kiss ass or have an attitude.

Now Todd's in *Vogue* and the gossip columns all the time and even has his own segment on Cindy Crawford's *House of Style* show on MTV. He gives practical fashion tips to the audience, like thrift-store shopping and how models stuff their bras. Todd's been creating things for women forever. He made felt purses for all the cool girls in second grade.

I'm sitting on the floor backstage at Todd's trippy

*Billy Beyond
and Todd Oldham
by Roxanne Lowit*

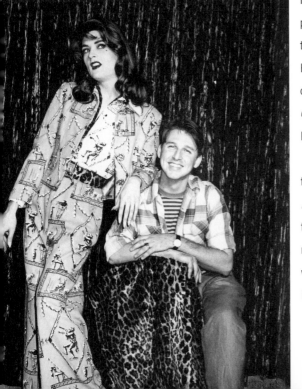

show, a "windows to the soul" voyage to India and Morocco. Todd's assistant, Angel, is smiling and handing out colored metal crucifixes that Todd made.

Christy Turlington has just finished getting some sparkles on her face. Christy, Kate Moss, Billy Beyond, and nine other girls are getting made up, bewigged, and sparkled.

Christy in profile has a warm, calming beauty. The Metropolitan Museum uses her face as a mold for their mannequins. Dorothy is in love with her big lips.

The hardest-working person backstage is Kevyn Aucoin, the makeup artist. He's got an unlisted phone number and hangs out with movie stars.

Once Kevyn completes their looks, the models don't have much to do until the show starts, so Christy and her friends sit cross-legged on the floor, smoking cigarettes, drinking champagne from plastic glasses, and talking about guys.

The rule for writers backstage is: No talking to the models. I'm relieved, because I'm not sure what there is to ask. "Um, Christy, what's it like to have your face in the museum?" Or, "Kate, did Kevyn do a good job on your makeup?" Or, "What's your favorite fabric tonight?" If a supermodel has something interesting to say, there are TV shows and publishers ready to listen. But in the world of beauty, there are times to shut up and let the beauty speak for itself. I want to look relevant, so I keep writing this in my notebook, again and again.

Todd's designs are so funky that I wonder who other than a model could pull them off: a blazer with mirrors, a fake leather pantsuit. Todd says he designs for women who are free-thinking and comfortable in their own skin.

I see a middle-aged woman wearing Oldham, a navy blue skirt with many different colored stones attached to it. She must be comfortable in her skin because she pulls it off.

It turns out to be Todd's mother. Mrs. Oldham has a Southern accent and is talking to Elsa Klensch, the white-faced black-haired lady who hosts CNN's *Style* TV show. "Well, hey, Miz Klensch, can I get you some champagne or an apple?"

All the fashion people watch Elsa. She's one of those cool Gloria Swanson–like women who gay guys imitate behind her back but are sincere when they are deferential in her presence.

"Sometimes when we see Todd on TV we're like Gomer Pyle," says Mrs. Oldham. "We just say, 'Golllll-y.' We never thought he'd be this big."

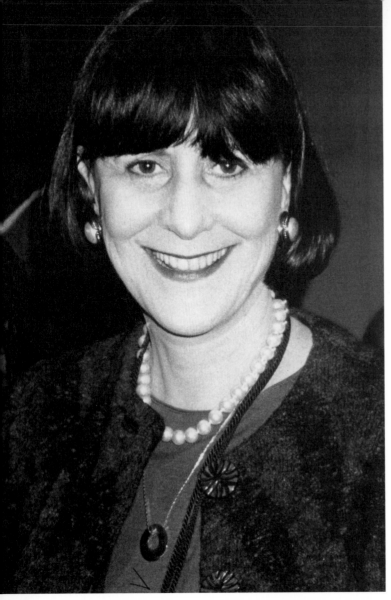

Elsa Klensch
by Roxanne Lowit

She says Todd wasn't obsessed with beauty growing up; he was more interested in figuring out how things worked.

A few feet away from us there's a beautiful woman with giant cheekbones and a lint brush. She has one of those round Debbie Harry kind of faces. I'd take her picture, but I didn't bring a camera. Her body is short and voluptuous, the sort that Rubens painted in the seventeenth century. So why is this woman taking the lint off Kate Moss's "mystic mosaic suit" instead of walking down the runway?

Relative fleshiness is valued when it reflects wealth and health. In Western society today, it symbolizes sloth and poor health. This will not change unless there's a famine or it somehow turns out that a breakfast of bacon, sausage, and buttered toast dunked in egg yolk is nutritious.

But again, why can't we celebrate more women who are undeniably beautiful but not extra-tall-and-thin model clones? This is because most of us get our visions of beauty not from museums, but from advertisements. (Though the best ad work will probably be in museums generations from now.) Contemporary beauty is about selling products, clothing especially. And most clothes hang better on tall, thin women. This is not to say that fashion-world beauty is the only kind that exists, but it is the only kind that they can be expected—as business people—to put forth, including renegades like Todd Oldham. In other words, don't expect new standards of beauty on the runway, only new models.

And even if we were going to contemporary art museums by the busload, we wouldn't be seeing different approaches to beauty. Whether or not you like the art of recent years, it's reasonable to say it's more about sex, politics, and darkness than beauty in repose.

So those of us eager to see new visions of beauty don't need to trash the fashion world, we just have to keep looking everywhere and elsewhere.

Mrs. Oldham looks at Christy Turlington and Kate Moss and smiles. "Now we all know that lasting beauty is what's inside," she says. "But it's astounding the gift that these girls were given."

4

anybody—skinny or not—is welcome to join Tiny Burgess's Modeling Club at Dwight Morrow, a mostly black high school in Englewood, New Jersey. Tiny is a God-given name, not a nickname, but the students call her Ms. Burgess.

Ms. Burgess teaches biology, but once a week after school, her "babies," her "favorite people"—twelve girls and four boys—have gotten together to learn the proper posture for tonight's fashion show. Mr. Hurley, the shop teacher, has built an Astroturf-colored runway just for tonight and set it up in the cafeteria.

The cafeteria is decorated with pink and purple bunting, balloons, and candelabras. The folding chairs are unfolded. Ms. Burgess, the hostess and emcee, sounds more like Don Cornelius than a biology teacher tonight. But she doesn't have Mr. Cornelius's playlist, so she lets one of the young people DJ. "The teens know what's popular," she says.

I drove to New Jersey tonight with the photographer Corinne Day—who will shoot the show for *Interview*—and her assistant. It's for an article about the popularity of modeling.

Corinne, twenty-eight, discovered Kate Moss, the waif in the Calvin Klein ads. Kate's become a supermodel and she's still a teenager. She's helped to sell many pairs of underwear but has upset a lot of feminists. They write "Feed me" on her Calvin Klein posters. "You can't be healthy and look like

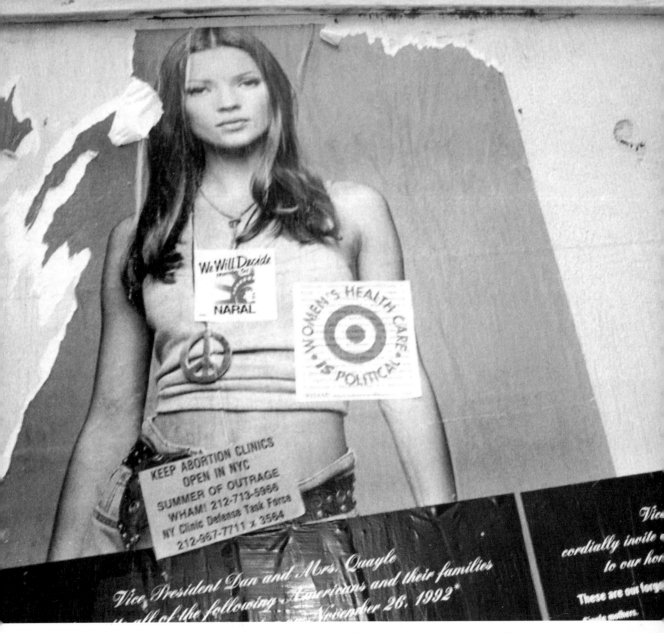

*Kate Moss
by Sandra-Lee Phipps*

that," feminists say. "It's the concentration camp look.... For every step
forward women make, there's a backlash."

Corinne had no idea that Kate, her muse, was upsetting people. Besides,
she says, Kate has never been imprisoned and she doesn't starve herself.
She eats tons.

Corinne has a little-girl voice, straight blond hair, translucent skin, and
some darkness under her eyes. She wears black socks with white Converse
sneakers, black jeans, and a pullover. She's from Ickenham, England. She

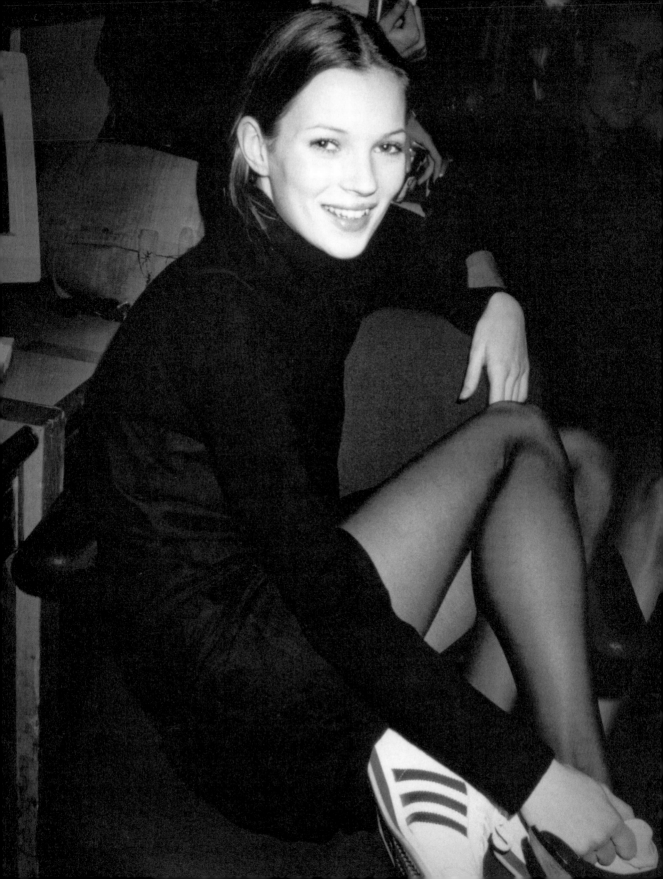

used to model but got bored and became a photographer for *The Face.* Corinne saw Kate and fell in love. That's how Kate's career started. She was *The Face*'s first model mascot. Kate is Corinne's ideal: skinny, young, unaffected, sweet. The va-va-voom models don't work for her.

When Corinne was a teenager, she was extra skinny like Kate. People used to tease her for being shaped like a pencil. "I hated my body and used to wear layers and layers of clothes to cover myself up." She ate and ate but was still bone thin. "I probably felt the same way a fat girl would." She was beaten up in high school until she learned to throw a punch and got some respect.

The people who trash skinny models, Corinne says, "are probably middle-aged women who started to put on weight—like all humans do—whenever they got past the age of twenty-five and have forgotten that there are a lot of skinny teenagers. They are making a big deal out of nothing. Clothes just happen to look really brilliant on thin people."

There's hip-hop and R&B in the background as Ms. Burgess, dressed in all white and a Sunday go-to-meeting hat, introduces each young person's entry onto the runway: "Beauty, brains, and poise bring tall, attractive Judy Joseph to the runway…. Her sign is my sign and that sign is Pisces…. Judy plays the flute in the band and attends the Barbizon School of Modeling. She would like to be a professional model and designer and, well, folks, she has the height, the look, and the know-how. Put them together and you're looking at success." Judy is wearing bell-bottom pants, a midriff blouse, a midnight-blue vest, and platform shoes.

"And she wears it oh so well," says Ms. Burgess.

Ms. Burgess enunciates each student's name, sign, dream, and wardrobe as smooth as a professional radio voice: Esmeralda Almanzar, Melina Medina, Peaches Smith, Pooran Sookoo….

"She's workin' it," the crowd says of Ms. Burgess. "She's dope."

Ms. Burgess has to be the friendliest teacher I've ever

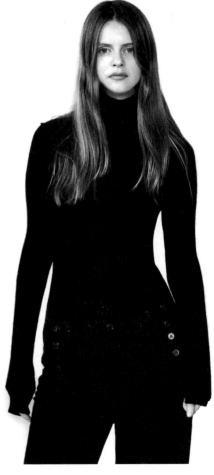

LEFT: *Kate Moss by Roxanne Lowit*

BELOW: *Corinne Day, courtesy of Corinne Day*

seen. I want to invite her over for supper or at least bake her a cake. Maybe if she'd been my biology teacher, I would have better mastered the reproductive system of the worm and made higher than a D.

But then again, I spent biology class sitting in the back, hunched over, my legs shaking up and down, hoping I'd make it through the day without being called "sooo groooss" or "monster face." Any kind of reproductive system was the last thing on my mind.

High school was when I learned that a homely face can be despised on sight and that beauty was the most instantly recognizable and pleasing trait a human could possess.

Even today, when I go to the Gap or Met Food and have a pretty teenager for a cashier, I look down as I hand her my cash.

Although my high school tormentors may have been guilty of what Truman Capote called the one unforgivable sin—deliberate cruelty—they were speaking the truth. The hallways of high school may be the only courtroom of beauty harsher than a three-way-mirror in a fluorescently lit dressing room.

But tonight, nobody's getting mocked. That's because the show is being held at night—not during school hours—and there are more family members in the audience than students. And even though they're welcome, no fat or broken-out pupils joined the modeling club. There are times when it makes sense to lay low, sweet as Ms. Burgess is.

A baby crawls onto the runway. "Don't knock my baby down!" a mother shouts. No babies are stepped on, but sometimes I see a price tag on a garment. The clothes fit fine. Ms. Burgess's girlfriend donated some of her own designs, and so did Dante Tuxedos of Teaneck.

"Fashions may come and fashions may go," says Ms. Burgess, "but the jeans world has been around for a long time and I believe it's here to stay—as Peaches and Melina show jeans—stonewashed jeans, jeans with patches, jeans with jackets. It's a jeans world, and if you don't believe it ask a teen and she will tell you: 'I prefer jeans.'

"And they wear them *oh so well*." Everybody says that part together now.

When the show ends, each model stands on the green runway holding a red rose. Ms. Burgess tells each "parent or guardian" to come to the runway

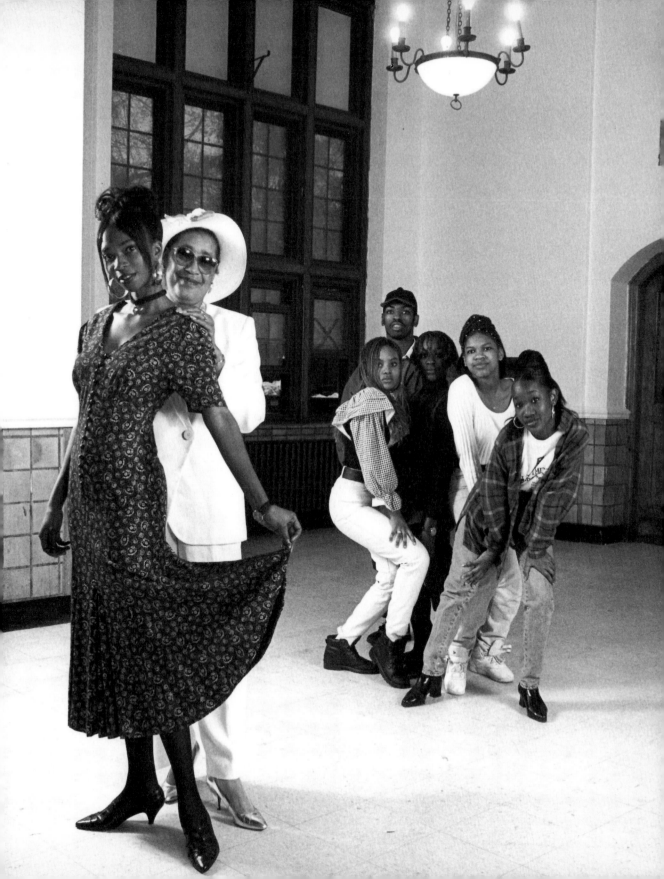

and receive a rose from his or her child. Then the models, all in their formal wear, stand in a line outside a classroom to get their pictures taken by Corinne. They tell me that their favorite models are Cindy Crawford and Naomi Campbell, and they know them mostly from TV.

Ms. Burgess goes first. She and her "babies" are so happy that it would be a drag, maybe even a little mean, to ask her about feminist theories on modeling.

"When the youngsters came out on the runway, I got goose bumps. They looked gorgeous. When we started practicing, I could hardly get them to walk down the runway.

"I don't advise young people on professional modeling," Ms. Burgess continues as Corinne clicks. "I don't know about that." Besides, most of the kids want to be psychologists, not models. "These youngsters are relatively shy and not as shy afterward. Peaches Smith was so shy last year, she's just blossomed. . . . If a heavy girl came in, I would encourage her. If she wants to model, undoubtedly she has something about herself that she feels good about and I should improve on that. Our club is fun and it gets kids to work together."

Corinne thinks all the kids are sweet. Her favorite, though, is not one of the models. He's a Latin boy, maybe fourteen years old. His girlfriend, Elba, is having her picture taken. He's just watching. You can see why he's Corinne's type: thin, smooth skin, angel face, bashful.

"Can I take your picture?"

Corinne shoots and shoots and the boy laughs and laughs. It's like Corinne is tickling him with the camera.

"One more," she says. "Take off your cap."

One shot.

"That's it," the boy says. He puts his hand in Elba's. They say good-bye to Ms. Burgess and walk down the hallway. They'll see her in class on Monday.

It was the kind of high school moment that Dorothy and I talk about. It's beauty and youth, and much of the beauty of youth is its purity and unaffectedness. Elba and her boyfriend don't know what their looks do to other people, don't know that the photographer was saying "how beautiful."

"I just want this night to be a great memory for them," says Ms. Burgess.

One of my favorite photographers is Bruce Weber. People ask him about beauty all the time. "I always think of that wonderful part in *Julia*," he once said, "where Vanessa Redgrave walks across the lawn and Jane Fonda looks at her and says at this time in her life she was the utmost of her beauty and it would never happen again." When these moments are photographed, "these [people] can show their grandchildren and say, 'Look at the way I looked. Wasn't I special?'"

"This is why we're hung up on this whole beauty trip," I once told Dorothy. "We still haven't gotten over not being in one of those photographs ourselves."

5

it was only two days ago that Judy Joseph had modeled in her high school cafeteria. Today, she's graduating from the Barbizon School of Modeling. The ceremony's at the Holiday Inn in Hasbrouck Heights, New Jersey, right off the turnpike and next to McDonald's. Judy's with Obie, her mother, and Jane, her sister. Her dad is out of town on business.

Charlotte Thompson in the model stance by Michel Delsol

We're in the cocktail lounge. The only food for sale is fried cheese. Everyone passes and has an orange juice. Obie tells me that she was first runner-up in the Miss African National Bank (Nigeria) pageant before Judy was born. But when Obie's father found out she was cavorting with beauty queens, he said no more. She couldn't show herself off on a platform because that was a sure way to get banged up.

Obie says that Judy has been interested in fashion since she was knee high to a duck. She's always wanted to model. "She was always messing with her dresses, looking in the mirror." Now Judy wants the same thing her mother did: to be publicly recognized for her beauty. "Wherever she goes, I go with her," Obie says.

The banquet room is filled with parents holding cameras. It's a cross between a bar mitzvah without the booze and food and a high school football game. A troubadour who has won the titles Mr. Talent America, Mr. Teen New Jersey, and Mr. Black New Jersey has on a tuxedo with a lime bow tie and sings "This Is the Most Important Day of My Life." He bows his head and ponders during the pretaped instrumental parts.

Forty perky and cute girls and one self-possessed boy, aged from seven to seventeen, come out and say, "Hello, my name is...." Besides modeling, makeup, and poise tips, Barbizon also teaches table manners. They do not

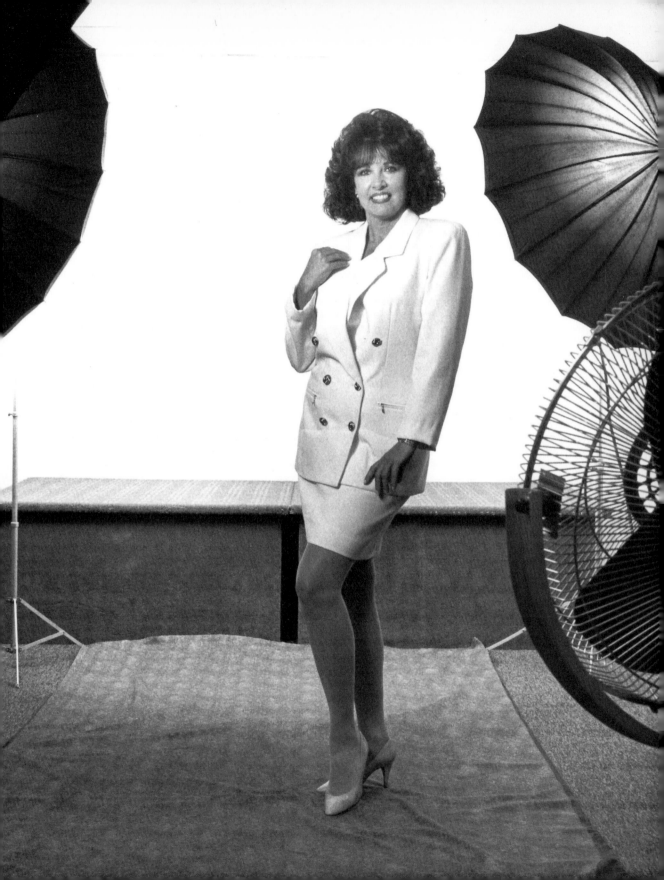

perform any "don't eat your peas with a knife" skits, but they do mime, mannequin, and vogue to Michael Jackson and Madonna songs. Two of the most embarrassing moments of my life were (1) when I was cornered at a street festival by a mime, and (2) when I walked in on a friend voguing in his living room. But here I'm not embarrassed because the Barbizon graduates are not self-conscious. This is pure suburban teen glamour and they are all proud and poised. Parents wave with one hand and take pictures with the other as their children take a few steps on the two-foot runway.

The man videotaping "this priceless event I'm sure you'll cherish" hands his video cam to an assistant and introduces himself. He's been in "the fashion, pageant, and cosmetic industries for almost two decades." In addition to selling the Barbizon videotapes, he's in charge of the Miss New Jersey World competition. He sounds just like Richard Simmons. "I see a lot of great careers here, I really do. Parents, get behind your kids a hundred and ten percent."

Afterward, back in the cocktail lounge, I meet Charlotte Thompson, who runs Barbizon in these parts of New Jersey. Ms. Thompson has been with Barbizon for twenty years and has also modeled. She was on the cover of *Miss Executive Female* in 1979. She's in all white, including heels, with a big head of copper-brown hair and expertly applied makeup. Through most of the ceremony, she stood in the model stance. "The model stance gives you a line and it's very professional."

Ms. Thompson never pauses when she talks about Barbizon. She could be on a company cassette. I ask her about "the great career opportunities" that await her graduates.

"Our greatest contribution is making them more poised, more aware of themselves. They come in shaking, looking down at the floor. We're there for confidence and polish. Now they can walk into any room—whether it's McDonald's or college—and feel better about themselves. The stigma of Barbizon is that we guarantee success for everybody, and if that doesn't happen then it's our fault, we're a rip-off."

"Would you ever turn anyone away?" I ask.

"No [even senior citizens are welcome], because of the commercial aspects, Ken. Everybody has some possibility, maybe for fragrance promotion." Fragrance promotion means standing poised and confident in a department store while spritzing consumers with perfume.

On her way out of the bar, Ms. Thompson slips her card to the bartender. He's got the smooth face of a teen dream date but also has biceps and is old enough to legally serve alcohol cocktails.

"Have you ever considered a career in modeling?"

6

if you're cursing Barbizon while squirting angry Bloomingdale's shoppers with perfume, maybe you should have listened to Eileen Ford to begin with. The Ford Modeling Agency's number is listed in the Manhattan directory, and the rules are laid down in its recording: "Ford holds interviews for young girls five-foot-nine and over and between the ages of fourteen and nineteen."

I get Mrs. Ford on the line. "Mrs. Ford, a book about beauty would be incomplete without you."

"What if I die?" she asks.

I'm in the Ford waiting room, the only person who is not a beautiful teenager. God, I hope they don't think I'm trying to model. Just because he had a notion to be nasty, a friend of mine once shouted to me as he was getting off a crowded bus: "Sorry you didn't get that modeling job."

"Bless that poor young man's heart," I knew the other passengers were thinking. "He believes he can be a model."

Mrs. Ford can see me now.

She is seventy and looks younger. She wears Chanel with no hose. Her red nails are so sharp I wish I had an itch. She sits with her legs curled back on the seat of her chair.

Mrs. Ford has been the queen of the modeling world since the 1940s.

She is as straightforward as she can be, no attitude, no Stepford wife. She's glad to answer questions, but not interested in having a Platonic dialogue about beauty. It's a lot more simple than you writers think, she says. Her beauty rules are not subject to debate.

Mrs. Ford says modeling is all about money. Her concern is not the general public, but her clients. Her job is finding the appropriately beautiful model for each client.

Besides money, modeling is about creating a dream. "Women want to see things they can dream about and inspire to better themselves. You want to dream you can get a [certain] dress. Women are much better off today, you know, things are much less expensive."

What the model is like, what the model's family background is, doesn't matter. "What counts is what the girl does in front of a camera."

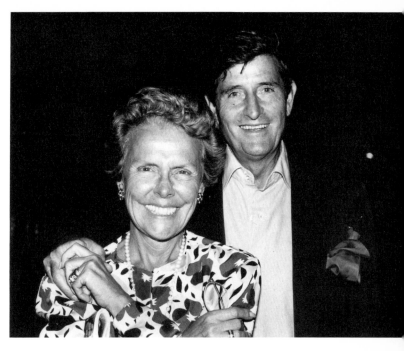

*Eileen and Jerry Ford
by Roxanne Lowit*

Models, unlike actresses, don't pose a threat to women because, says Mrs. Ford, they are not sexually available to men. Men do not read fashion magazines.

Models make women feel great. Period. Mrs. Ford has not heard about the anger over waif models.

Some cosmetic surgery is okay, but not all. Mrs. Ford has had silicone injected into her face for eliminating wrinkles. It says so in her book, *Beauty Now and Forever*. She says she'd have more work done if she had the time. She'd have liposuction but says she's too old. She draws the line at breast implants and tanning in the nude.

Mrs. Ford does not think about male beauty, even though the Ford male models are just down the staircase. Her husband, Jerry, loves her and that's enough. But she once said if he left her she'd "kill him."

She says the worst part of her job is rejecting people, and the best part is making beautiful young girls feel secure. Some of the girls live with the Fords. She doesn't fantasize about turning ugly ducklings into swans. Her job is to turn swans into paid swans.

"I took a fifteen-year-old girl to the hairdresser the other day. Her hair was so kinky it took two hours to straighten. The girl said to me, 'I've never been able to run my fingers through my hair before. I want everybody to see my beautiful hair.'" Mrs. Ford smiles.

When Mrs. Ford says this I realize how easy it is to mock anyone who talks about beauty but isn't as eloquent as Oscar Wilde. That's why Mrs. Ford gets described in some articles as a mean and superficial rich lady.

But the business of beauty is inherently superficial, cold, and exclusive. The nonbeautiful make a mistake if we look to it for promises or reassurances about our own looks. Mrs. Ford doesn't even pretend to be interested in hiring normal-looking models the "everyone is beautiful in his or her own way" people clamor for. To pay an average-looking model would be, in her eyes, rewarding mediocrity. She would be acting like the Communist skating judge in Peter Morris's Cold War–era poem, "Communist Ice Show":

> It's been an easy day. I feel like a judge at a Communist
> ice-show, giving perfect scores to clumsy Bulgarians while
> penalizing the British for executing flawless pirouettes.

When I see photos of Mrs. Ford's past and present models (Suzy Parker, Jane Fonda, Carmen, Lauren Hutton, Candice Bergen, Isabella Rosselini, Christy Turlington...), I think the same things I did at Todd Oldham's show: The best models *are* extraordinary-looking, not the product of airbrushers. And beauty does not have to cheapen when it becomes business.

I want to say we should develop more refined ways to show beauty, but perhaps it isn't possible. I picture Hutton by Avedon, Carmen by Horst, and Christy Turlington walking down a runway, and can't think of alternatives, can't think of a better way to present contemporary beauty. There's no need to apologize for the best of our pop culture; we ought to cherish it.

7

arthur Elgort says I can come by his studio and watch him shoot Naomi Campbell for *Vogue*.

Arthur smokes a pipe. He has glasses and a little bit of hair. He's been working for *Vogue* since the seventies. Arthur's charming but not affectedly so. He puts everyone in his presence at ease.

Arthur kisses Naomi when she walks in. She's got lips like sugar, the Echo and the Bunnymen song goes. Her skin glows and it's before makeup. White teeth, clear eyes. Naomi often has straight black hair that extends almost to her navel, but today she's got a pixie cut.

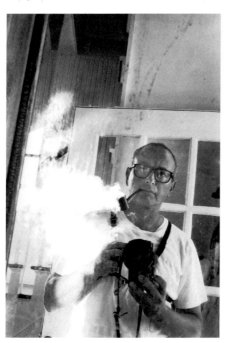

*Arthur Elgort
self-portrait*

"Would you like cappuccino or tea?" Arthur asks Naomi. "I'll give you a choice, sweetie. What appeals to ya?" Arthur sounds like a butcher from Brooklyn, giving the finest cuts to his favorite customer. He admits he's a bit like a horse doctor, always examining women's legs and teeth.

"It's spring and Naomi is doing it all over again, making people fall in love with her, the way it's been done for thousands of years. And she's beautiful, just like a flower or bird," Arthur says.

Naomi's posing with two other models today—Beverly Peele and another model. I don't know her name but she's from Somalia. While Naomi waits to be made up, she flips through an Italian *Vogue* and points out her friends such as Helmut Newton. Naomi's so famous that everybody knows about her dates. She used to go out with Robert De Niro, but now she's engaged to Adam Clayton, the bassist from U2.

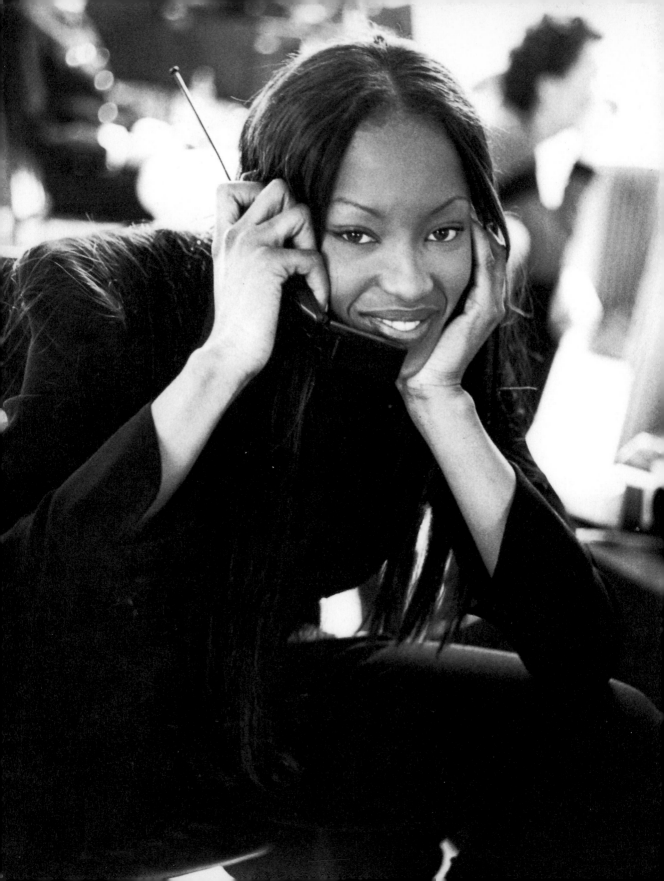

There's a biography of her coming out, and she's trying to have it killed. The author says he's scared when he walks the streets of New York. Naomi's friends spit on him. I remember reading that Marilyn Monroe told Truman Capote that lots of men would be glad to murder for her.

Naomi has lip-synched in videos to Michael Jackson and George Michael songs, but I read in a magazine that she can sing in her own voice.

"Um, when is your album coming out?" I ask her.

"Soon," she says.

Naomi sprawls out on a white couch. She's so confident and calm, she makes Arthur feel good. "The Queen of Sheba," he calls her. If beauties have become the new royals, it's because they've outlasted everyone else, Arthur says.

The portable phone in Naomi's bag rings and she asks someone to get it. There are plenty of people to oblige. For this one photo shoot there are: *Vogue* editor Phyllis Posnick and her assistant, two makeup artists, a hair stylist, and Arthur's two assistants (not including his three associates in the back of the loft who administrate his photos and his life). It must be the man from U2 on the phone; Naomi whispers and smiles. As she talks on the phone, Arthur shoots her. This is how he gets some of his best shots: spontaneous and unplanned. That's how he got one of his favorites, the shot of Christy Turlington in a Paris café. The shoot had ended, and she and Arthur went out for some *pomme frites* and champagne. He brought his camera and captured a moment of beauty and believable grandeur.

When he tells me the story of that photo, I can see why he prefers to work alone with a model. But part of the reason he's so loved at *Vogue* and has lasted so long is that he's an obliging man. He snubs no one, not even the assistants. If *Vogue* sends over a model who's not his type, he'll find a way to appreciate her. If big-boned women with nose rings are hot next season, Arthur will find a way to "dig" them, even if he doesn't fall in love.

"Fall in love?" Well, Arthur really means enchanted by, smitten with. The kind of girl you want to have a "cup of tea" with when a shoot's over.

That kind of beauty, says Arthur, the kind that moves you, is defined by your past—the first boy or girl you kissed, the first movie star you had a crush on.

Naomi Campbell by Arthur Elgort

OVERLEAF: *Christy Turlington by Arthur Elgort*

49

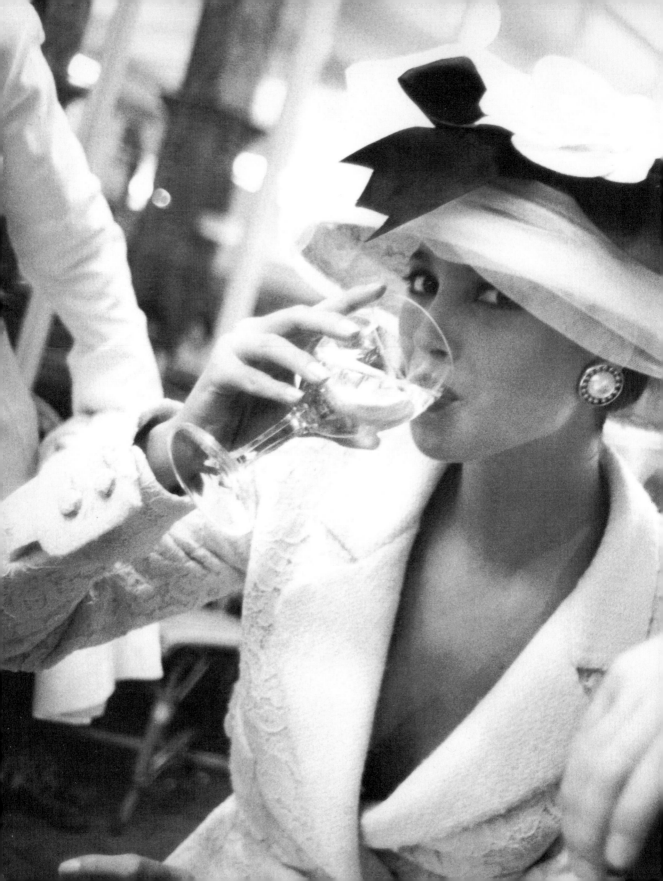

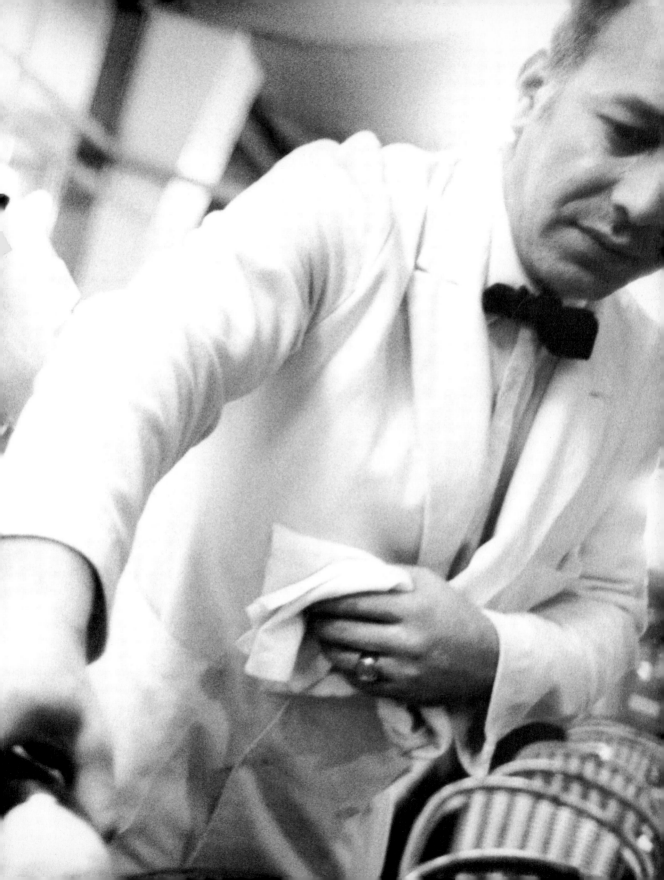

I think Arthur is right. And here's another reason why it can be embarrassing to talk about beauty, and adolescent-sounding when we do, especially as we get older: A lot of the beauty trip—whether it's lingering over Arthur's photographs or getting your face changed—is an attempt to re-create, or at least be reminded of, youthful romance.

And romance has a lot to do with youth and beauty. It happens when two people are young enough and attractive enough to fall in love with each other on sight. Of course, romance exists for the aging and the homely, but the ugly truth is that it doesn't happen as much and isn't as photogenic when it does.

My roommate in college had also been my best friend in high school. He was fat and I had zits, so we didn't get invited to parties or date that much. But it wasn't so bad. We could make each other laugh and we both liked Blondie and the Sex Pistols.

Then one summer he lost weight, but my face didn't clear up. Our friendship didn't change at first, but the way strangers treated him did. We'd go to parties and still find the most remote corner wall to lean against. But now he'd almost instantly be drawn into the center of the room and eventually to someone's bed. I'd still be leaning, peeling the label off my beer bottle, and rolling it into sticky little balls.

I realized not much later that I, too, had fallen for him. It was the first time I had fallen in love. And when I was spurned in the end, he pointed to the mirror.

"Take a look at yourself," he said.

I've been doing that ever since, correcting as much as I can while still longing for his type—pretty boys with smooth skin and black hair.

Arthur's type, ever since he was a little boy, has been ballerinas and dancers. He falls for them to this day.

True love, says Arthur, is the way he feels for his wife and two kids. And yes, his wife is his type.

"What does your wife think about your working with beautiful women every day?"

"My wife is a self-possessed and busy person who has a much more important job than I have as far as she's concerned." She develops and directs operas. But Arthur doesn't make it difficult for her. "I don't come home and say, 'Honey, you should have seen the legs on Naomi today.'"

Beautiful women come to his studio every day wanting his approval. Does he ever mess around? It isn't a temptation, Arthur says, because the girls never fall for him. He's more of an uncle or older brother. "The girls don't look at me and gasp and say, 'Look at that guy. I'd like to jump him and have fun with him for a while.' It was not my lot in life to be the kind of guy who walks in a bar and have people want to buy me a drink." Things would be different, Arthur says, if he looked like a young Marcello Mastroianni.

The photo shoot is over in an hour. The girls had spent more time in makeup and hair. They all kiss Arthur good-bye.

As demanding as the models' schedules can be, there's something simple about all of this. "The minimum any model has to do is show up. Someone's gonna get them cappuccino or tea, tell them how lovely they are, set everything up. As long as they get themselves here, they're still a contender."

None of Arthur's *Vogue* work is on the walls of this enormous white loft, only his portraits of jazz greats and cowboys. He never gets bored with beauty, but is happier when photographing his favorite musicians. Arthur's still daydreaming, though, about Natasha Richardson, the actress. He'd seen her in an O'Neill play the night before he shot her. She is his ideal subject—a talented beauty.

People don't always tell the truth about how they deal with beauty, especially to strangers in the daytime. And for all I know Arthur is courting aspiring models in a suite at the Plaza every chance he gets. Not that I'd blame him if he is, but I think he's being straight with me. And at the risk of sounding naive, I look at him as a guide, as someone whose embrace of and access to beauty leads not to smug arrogance or lechery, but to the first step in a ladder leading to something far greater.

8

kristen McMenamy is the model who says she looks like a Martian drug addict. She's chopped off most of her hair and all of her eyebrows. So she's used to being stared at.

Now she's lying—stomach down and topless—on a couch in the dressing room of a New York City nightclub. She's cohosting an AIDS benefit with Miss America, Leanza Cornett. Kristen is surrounded by courtiers: me, Dorothy, a publicist, makeup people, photographers, and Bob Morris, a columnist for the *New York Times.*

We all can see Kristen's breasts because the makeup girls are painting red AIDS ribbons down the middle of Kristen's naked back. Miss America wore a red ribbon on her breast the night she was crowned and has made AIDS aware-ness the duty of her reign.

"I always wanted to be Miss America," says Kristen. "I always watched those beauty contests. They were my bible. But I could never win because I didn't have that Miss America smile or those Miss America answers."

But when she goes backstage to meet Miss America, Kristen, a head taller, is the one who is mobbed by photographers. I'd always fantasized about being sur-rounded by paparazzi. This is the closest I'll get. Miss America, who used to be the Little Mermaid at Disney World, returns to a corner, alone with her chaperone.

Kristen had always given Dorothy hope. "Damn that girl's ugly," Dorothy had thought. "If she can model, so can I." But when she sees Kristen in the flesh, Dorothy changes her mind. Like all supermodels, Kristen is tall, poised, thin, has great skin, and isn't close to thirty yet. A photo can make her look goofy, especially when she chooses to have a facial seizure in front of the camera. But if she really wanted to, Kristen could be a conventional model clone. Before not having eyebrows made her shine, she was a normal model getting so-so jobs.

"She radiates energy," says Dorothy. "She looked at me from on high." This is the power of the model, of beauty: You can get a nonsexual high from just being in its presence.

"This could happen only in New York or Los Angeles," I say. "If Kristen and Miss America met anywhere else in America, I guarantee Kristen would have been the one alone in a corner." I remember a letter to the editor in *Vogue* where a lady from Idaho said Kristen frightened her. But Manhattan is filled with people like Dorothy and me, people who moved here in part to get away from the perky suburban prettiness that had no place for us. Tonight, gawky urban glamour triumphed.

"Yeah, Kristen was probably real gawky in high school," says Dorothy. "I wish there had been a beauty like her when I was a teenager. Maybe Kristen will help create a legacy. Boneheads and misfits can aspire to beauty and glamour."

"But don't look to models for confirmation about your looks," I say. "It's great if you see yourself reflected in their beauty, but that's not their job. They get paid to be goddesses, not role models."

Kristen NcMenamy
by Roxanne Lowit

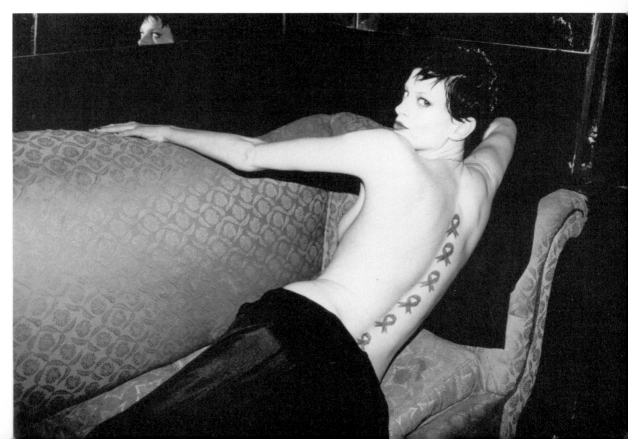

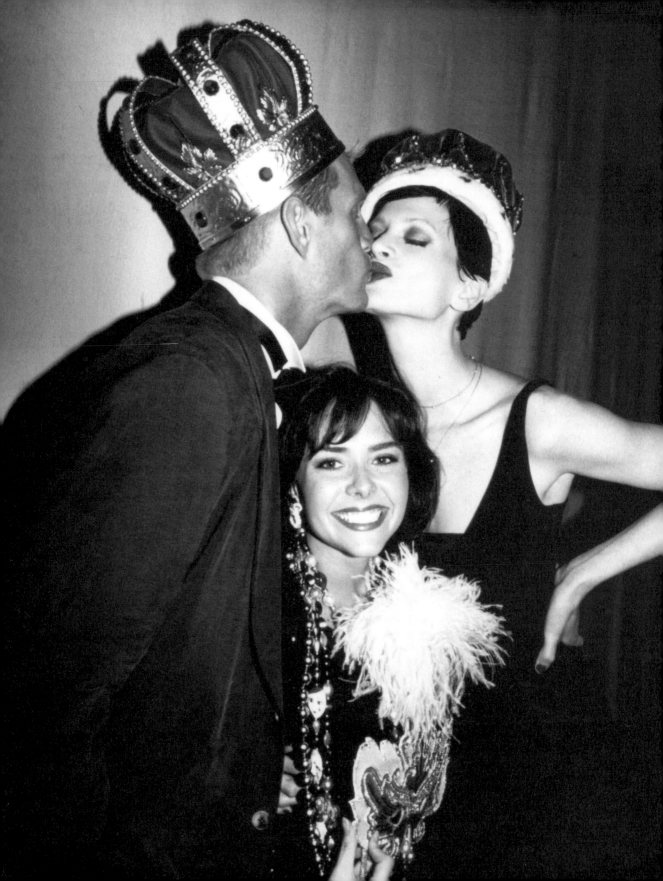

Miss America is as gracious as she can be. She isn't allowed to be as spacey as Kristen. For one thing, she's a public AIDS spokesperson. For another, she's representing a corporation, the Miss America Organization. There's even a CEO. That's why she always has a chaperone at her side.

Leanza says she keeps her feet on the ground by talking to her parents every night. She'll try to make it on Broadway or in TV when her reign is over.

I tell Dorothy I saw Leanza once before, the night she was crowned in Atlantic City.

The boardwalk was filled with families wearing buttons with pictures of their state-anointed beauty queens. The adults reminded me of parents who shout real loud at Little League games. Hanging in hotel lobbies were high school graduation-style portraits of the contestants who slept there. I heard some of the maids fighting over who would get to change Miss Idaho's sheets.

The Miss America contestants all could have passed for airline stewardesses. I imagined their smiles staying in place even if a troublemaker stormed the stage and demanded a cocktail or almonds. I do not say this out of disrespect, because they were obviously talented to have gotten as far as they did. But the baked hair, caked makeup, forced smiles, and gowns better suited for a middle-aged woman named Toots than a college girl reminded me of a network-televised Barbizon graduation. This is why Miss America winners do not have photo shoots with Avedon, Horst, Weber, or Meisel after they win. The only Miss America still in vogue is the only one to have been dethroned, Vanessa Williams.

"They're all *Playboy* girls with their clothes on," says Dorothy. "Friendly and unthreatening. Easy-access American beauty."

"Do you realize how much better they'd look, though, if they had Mr. Kenneth or Oribe do their hair and shopped at Barney's?"

"You've lived in New York too long," Dorothy says. "Most of the country still loves those babes."

Dorothy says she's got her first *Playboy* flesh assignment. She's going to write the copy for the "Student Bodies" piece. I can go down south and hang out with two University of Georgia girls who'll be in the pictorial.

*Kristen McMenamy and
Miss America
by Roxanne Lowit*

9

two undergraduates from the University of Georgia are in Dorothy's "Student Bodies" pictorial: Amanda and Kelly. They're both seniors and both brunettes. They showed their breasts and pubic hair in *Playboy* and got to take home $500. The co-eds in the spread who didn't show pubic hair got just $250. Dorothy wrote the copy beneath their photos:

> "Amanda Roberts is a senior at the University of Georgia. While good looks run in the family—her mom was Miss Arkansas in the fifties—Amanda hopes to step to the other end of the lens and create 'erotic photography.' Georgia's Kelly Collins saves her highest praise for Mom. She studies family consumer science and journalism."

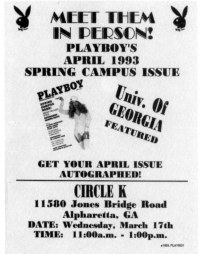

It's the day *Playboy*'s "Student Bodies" issue hits the newsstands. Kelly and Amanda are in the backseat of Don Donovan's car, a Cadillac sedan. Don is a regional marketing man for *Playboy;* he's driving the girls to autographings and radio interviews. Don is a gentle man who speaks slowly and with a Southern accent. Sometimes he gets a little flustered behind the wheel; he's from Texas and doesn't know all the Georgia roads. Amanda and Kelly help him out. Don's been working for *Playboy* for years, says they treat him right.

Don's taking the girls to Atlanta. They've just finished a signing at the college bookstore in Athens. Kelly's friends—mostly business majors in baseball caps—stood on one side of the store. Amanda's—

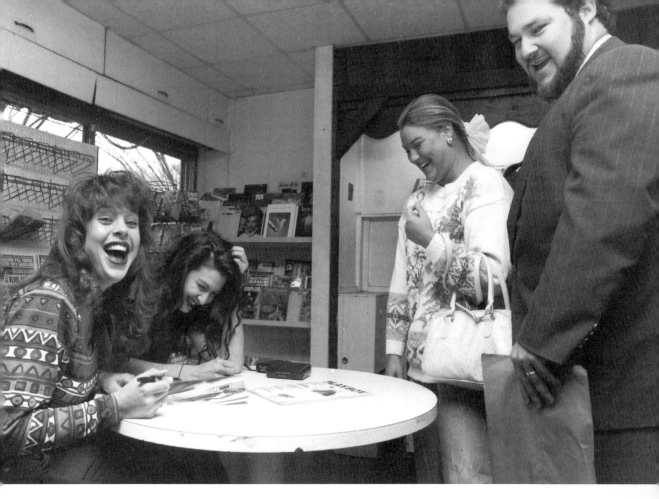

Kelly and Amanda
by Rochelle Campbell

all dressed in black, one with a mohawk—stood on the other. Amanda's boyfriend came by with roses and a card in the shape of the *Playboy* bunny.

Amanda and Kelly sat at a table by the window. College boys approached them bashfully for an autograph. Some boys on the sidewalk peeked in the window and smiled. "Y'all are beautiful," the boys said.

"Why, thank you."

Amanda pulled the plastic off the *Playboy*—"brand spankin' new." Amanda was on page 146 and Kelly on 147, so they autographed at the same time and the line went a lot quicker.

"Y'all don't cover up the artwork, now," one boy said.

Kelly changes into a proper white blouse, long blue skirt, and heels for her Atlanta appearances. Amanda puts on funky platform shoes and a black dress that reveals the Bauhaus tattoo on her back. She pulls a loose string off the back of Kelly's skirt as they enter the lobby of the radio station, morning drive rock. We're all met by the DJ, a man named Radical Bradford. He has an earring, beard, hair that's balding up front but long in the back, and wire-rimmed aviator glasses. He says hey to us all and stops suddenly to play air guitar when Skynard comes on.

They're on the air now, and the girls get asked the same questions they've been getting since word came out that they were *Playboy* posers.

"How did all this come about?"

Playboy came to campus, put an ad in the student paper. They set up at the Holiday Inn. Hundreds of girls tried out. *Playboy* took Polaroids of everyone and chose Amanda and Kelly. There were no feminist or religious protests, and *Playboy* was very professional.

"What did your parents think?"

Amanda doesn't talk to her parents. Kelly's parents weren't thrilled, but she wasn't cut off or anything.

"What do your boyfriends think?"

Amanda's boyfriend thinks it's great; he photographs her all the time. Kelly's boyfriend is okay about it, but feels kind of weird about having to share Kelly with millions of men.

"Why did you do this?"

Almost everyone on campus has already seen Amanda buck naked because she poses for art classes. She's also a photography major and hopes this is a way maybe to get a job at *Playboy* when she graduates. Kelly's friends saw the *Playboy* ad in the student paper and told her to go for it. Why not?

What Kelly really wants is a job in radio advertising. She's dressed the part. She'll graduate in a few months, so she talks to the station manager for a while. Don Donovan encourages her to write a follow-up letter when she gets home. But now we've got to get to the Circle K convenience store for an autograph session. Circle K sells gas, two hot dogs for ninety-nine cents, and more *Playboy*s than any chain in the country. Amanda and Kelly are in the backseat, checking their faces in Amanda's compact. It's pink and in the shape of a seashell. Kelly wears a lot more foundation.

They're talking about how much food they ate the night before. Ever since they posed for *Playboy*, they've been pigging out. When the PR stuff is finished tomorrow, they'll start watching themselves again. Kelly will go back to counting the number of calories in each M&M.

"I don't think any woman—even Cindy Crawford—is always happy with her looks," says Kelly.

Amanda and Kelly say they are always self-conscious and think they weigh too much.

"But if *Playboy* models are torturing themselves over five pounds, what about a Plain Jane or a girl who's getting mocked for her looks? What are they going through?" I ask.

"Hell," says Amanda. "A homely girl would think we're the most obnoxious and arrogant people in the world for talking about ourselves like this, but it's true."

Both Amanda and Kelly spend a lot of time adding and subtracting calories to figure out what they can eat. The more calories they burn on the StairMaster, the more baked potatoes they allow themselves. They spend time during class lectures computing calories. Kelly even has a notebook to keep track of it all. Exercise isn't fun or a release, it's just part of their beauty ritual.

There are as many vain people in gyms now as jocks. The two may look alike at first glance, but here's how to tell them apart: jocks get joy from exercise; vain people—like Kelly, Amanda, and me—do it because we'll feel worse if we don't. And because the tedium of working out twelve hours per week is preferable to the revulsion of seeing excess body fat in our mirrors.

It's not always easy to spot the true athlete in a gym. As long as I avoid aerobics classes and anything else that requires coordination, I can do my bicep curls and the StairMaster and pretend I'm a former high school jock. My pose will be shattered, though, if a guy approaches me because I'm real tall and says: "How 'bout shootin' some hoops with us?" Or, "Did you see the game last night?"

Um, which one?

Amanda's been dieting since she was twelve. She and her sister would fast for days before they went to the beach. The guys checked them out, so it was worth the hunger.

"Are y'all's boyfriends asking you to diet?" I ask.

"It's more a loathing thing," says Amanda, and Kelly nods. "The pressure is not coming from our boyfriends. Any guy who tries to force you to look a certain way is a jerk. We think our boyfriends are thinking about our weight, but they're usually not. Most guys can't tell the difference if we put on five pounds; they might not even notice until we gain twenty. But girls notice. It's really competitive."

Amanda says that whether girls admit it or not, they always want to be more attractive than their friends. Amanda and Kelly know that the other girls on campus are sizing them up, thinking, "Why did *they* get chosen?" It's like a female machismo—competition not based on athletics or money, but on beauty. But if competition is inevitable—who doesn't want to be beautiful?—why do you have to chastise yourself even when you're acknowledged to be the prettiest, like now?

"Once I reached my goal and I was my ideal weight, I freaked out," says Amanda. "I missed the longing. Everything falls back on beauty."

"Can't you acknowledge your beauty and go on to something else?"

"It's kind of like telling an alcoholic not to drink. This is not rational," says Amanda.

"What would happen if you could keep your looks but not think about them all the time?"

"I guess I'd feel better and be more aggressive.... But everything goes so much faster now. We're always seeing perfect bodies flashed in front of us. Kids in elementary school are wearing makeup and dieting. Five pounds may not be much, but it's also the fear of losing control, of gaining five pounds after that," says Amanda.

Amanda and Kelly's boyfriends aren't pretty boys, but both can be happy when they look in the mirror. They look at a photo of a shirtless Marky Mark, laugh, and crack open a beer. It's not a big deal for them to have a beer belly. Women are forgiving of men's bodies but not of each other's. It's the same things Dorothy talked about after Chippendale's. As long as women are seduced more by emotion and men more by looks, it will be ridiculous to expect equality on the beauty trip.

A bunch of pickup trucks are getting some self serve at the Circle K in

Alpharetta, a few miles outside Atlanta. The flyers in the window say: "Meet Them in Person. *Playboy*'s Spring Campus Issue. Get Your Issue Autographed." It's lunch hour, best dogs in the county and all the fixin's (serve yourself) are two for ninety-nine cents. Six Flav-o-Rich milk crates—three on each side—prop up a Formica tabletop. This is where Amanda and Kelly will sit and sign. The ice machine is hurling chunks non-stop. The customers, most of them in construction, are filling up their big ol' plastic cups. Free refills.

"How can they do this to us?" Amanda and Kelly are half kidding.

"Hot stuff," yells Debbie, the Circle K manager. She's just taken some chicken quesadilla out of the microwave and is carrying it to the counter, near the copies of *Playboy*. Debbie says some of the older cus-

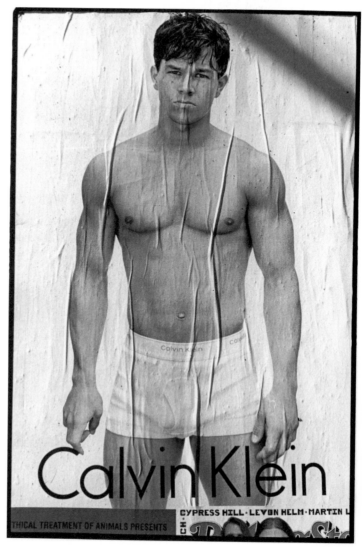

Marky Mark
by Michel Desol

tomers complained, so she put the *Playboy*s behind the counter. She smiles and says hey to Amanda and Kelly and gets a copy signed for her husband. "Shoot, if I'm gonna lose my husband, I'll lose him anyway. It won't be because of *Playboy*. Besides, these girls would leave him," she laughs.

Don Donovan is standing behind the girls as they sign their names, and two more men in suits join him. Ken Vaughn, regional sales, and a Circle K bigwig. "It's like an entertainment complex here," says Mr. Vaughn. "Get you some lunch, some entertainment, you're all set."

"That's right," says the Circle K man.

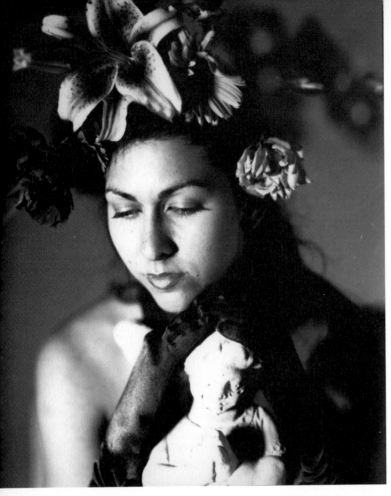

Amanda
by C. Jason Moore

"Did y'all get you some dogs?" the Circle K man asks the girls. "They're on the house."

"That's all right, thank you, though."

Most of the customers are Southern-gentlemen respectful to the girls. They say thank y'all, 'preciate it, and ask the same questions that were answered on the radio this morning. One man from Atlanta Gas and Light says to sign his copy "Eat me raw." The girls say no, uh-uh. "All right, then," he says.

Lunch hour's over, and Amanda and Kelly hug good-bye. Amanda and I are headed up to New York City, where she's going to do the *Montel Williams* TV show. (*Montel* preinterviewed both girls, and Amanda was more verbal.) Mr. Vaughn drives us to the airport. Don Donovan's got to drive Kelly to more autographings in Atlanta.

Amanda says that Kelly's really sweet, but they'd have never met if it hadn't been for posing for *Playboy*. She's sure Kelly and her friends would think she was a freak if they knew what she was really about.

Amanda whispers that she's afraid her nipple ring will set off the metal detector in the airport. She's the first girl in *Playboy* to be photographed wearing a nipple ring. She has other piercings, too—in her nose and vagina—but won't wear them while she's representing *Playboy,* at least not the nose ring.

When I was in college in the eighties, punk allowed plain and ugly people to become not beautiful, of course, but stylish. We'd shave our heads, pierce our ears a few times in the same lobe, wear tattoos and mascara, and guys like me could claim they were wearing foundation to look like Boy George, when it was really to cover up zits. To me, beauty has always meant nothing to hide, no flaws to conceal. So what's Amanda doing to her beauty?

Once we're on the plane and there are no *Playboy* people around, Amanda slams one back to calm her fear of flying and talks about her piercings and tattoo.

"It's fun to change my body," Amanda says. Traditional model beauty bores her. "Tattoos and piercings allow you to individualize yourself. You choose your own mark. To me, they're beautiful."

But I've spent my adult life trying to clear up my marks. "Anyway, isn't this more about mutilation than aesthetics?" I ask. "Isn't this very S/M?"

"Yes," says Amanda. She says it's a harsh beauty.

Tattoos and piercings instinctively attract the eye but can't create physical beauty. You can be fascinated by a beautiful tattoo while being otherwise oblivious to the person wearing it. And you can find someone stunningly beautiful and at the same time fantasize about tearing off their nose ring like a dry scab.

Amanda talks about the time she was a green–haired girl in Stephens County, Georgia. Her high school didn't know what to do with a girl who had a green mohawk. So they called her mother, the former Miss Arkansas, to make a deal. The school didn't have grounds to expel Amanda, though she had to be up to no good with a hairdo like that. She was just ugly to look at, the teachers said. So the principal told her mom that they would give Amanda a high school diploma if she left school and checked into an institution.

Charter Winds in Atlanta isn't really for crazy people; it's more the kind of place where rich parents put their kids when they're smoking too much weed and wrecking the family cars. Amanda was diagnosed as antisocial, but not anti-social enough to be under medication.

Amanda had to talk about her mother in therapy. She didn't know her mom was once Miss Arkansas until she was nine years old. She found out from her sister. All the photos and news clips and gowns were in the attic in boxes or mothballs. Her mom couldn't be an icon and a mother at the same time, so she banished all icons from the house. Amanda couldn't hang Duran Duran posters on her wall. It wasn't a religious thing; Jesus was forbidden, too.

Amanda's mom got up to three hundred pounds. She stayed home during family reunions; she didn't want to be compared to what she was. She doesn't wear makeup anymore, just tent dresses.

When Amanda left Charter Winds, she was in no mood to go home. She hitched to Los Angeles. She had no money and saw a sign at the Cavern on the Hollywood Strip: TOPLESS DANCERS NEEDED. The pay was okay, enough to get her a room to rent. But Amanda wanted to go to college and study photography. Her parents wouldn't pay tuition, so she moved to Athens, Georgia, got a dancing job, and put herself through school.

Amanda's role model became Betty Page, the hubba-hubba-bing-bang pin-up girl when Eisenhower was president. She was known as Miss Pinup of the World and the Queen of Bondage. Even today, guys get her tattooed on various body parts and read Betty Page fanzines. Betty had a full figure, long black hair, bangs (to shorten her forehead) and white skin. Amanda does favor her.

Amanda's voice is sweet and Southern. The tone is that of a Miss Arkansas responding to Bert Parks's questions. Only the words are different:

"With dancing, first you say, 'God, they asked me to work here, I must be pretty attractive.' Then it's the money. I make in a day what my boyfriend works hard to earn in a week. And there's freedom. You can sit around in your underwear and drink at the bar with your girlfriends. But after a while you get up there and you need a couple of drinks just to smile. The longer you're there, the more tainted you get. Your sexual side gets lost because you associate it with a job.

"My boyfriend is sweet and wonderfully supportive, but I really have to make it a point to be sexual with him sometimes.

"I've had offers [from classy joints] to dance after I graduate. There are very few people who can get out of dancing completely and get a 'legitimate' job. The good thing about dancing is you can go to almost any city and get a job that pays well. I'm grateful for it; it put me through school. But I really want to get a job in photography or at a magazine, though. I'm scared to see myself ten years down the line if I stay at this. There's a girl I work with now who has danced for twelve years and she's hollow, like a robot."

A car and a driver meet Amanda at the airport and take her to the *Montel Williams* TV studio in Times Square.

Dorothy and I sit in the *Montel Williams* greenroom, watching everything on a monitor. We're glad we're not sitting with the studio audience. It's a few minutes before the show starts and the producer is warming the crowd up, promoting cheerful stuff, like touching the shoulder of the person in front of you, shaking hands with your "neighbor next door." Dorothy and I do not like to touch strangers. We stayed indoors during Hands Across America.

"Do we have any singers in the audience?" the producer asks. A woman stands up and sings a Coke commercial, "I'd Like to Teach the World to Sing." There are many aspiring singers in New York. The audience doesn't know the topic of the show— *"Playboy's* Student Bodies." They're just glad to be on TV.

Four college girls from the "Student Bodies" pictorial are on the show tonight. Amanda, Doni from Central Michigan University, Jennifer from the University of Texas, and Marlee from Arizona State.

Montel Williams is a handsome, bald black man in his thirties, a former naval intelligence officer. *Montel's* publicist is in the greenroom, trying to convince Dorothy that Montel should be interviewed by *Playboy*.

Where's Amanda? The only student body in the greenroom is Marlee from Arizona State, who came with her mother. Marlee says she would have been five-foot-seven, but she had scarlet fever as a tyke, so now she's only five-five, and that limits her modeling options. She and her mom are glad you don't have to be tall to pose for *Playboy*. Marlee looks great, just like her photo, except now she's in a beige pants suit. Marlee's mom said the other girls are in wardrobe. Wardrobe? Marlee's mom said she wouldn't let her daughter change into anything; they'd spent a lot of time deciding on this outfit.

"You don't look sleazy enough. Let's get you into these."

That's what Montel's producer says to the three girls—Amanda, Jennifer, and Doni—who came alone, without their mothers. She hands them sequined outfits that Montel's wife—a former Vegas showgirl—has picked out for them. "I want to see some cleavage, goddamn," says Montel. "We've got ratings to think about."

The girls come out not looking like sexy co-eds, but disposable extras in a Vegas revue. Amanda had wanted to go out in her preferred all black with a red AIDS ribbon. They told her to take off the ribbon and put on a red sequined jacket. The girls' hairdos were floozied, giving them that whirly seventies look.

"They look awful!" Dorothy says. "Except for Marlee."

Montel Williams is the kind of talk show where the audience gets to do much

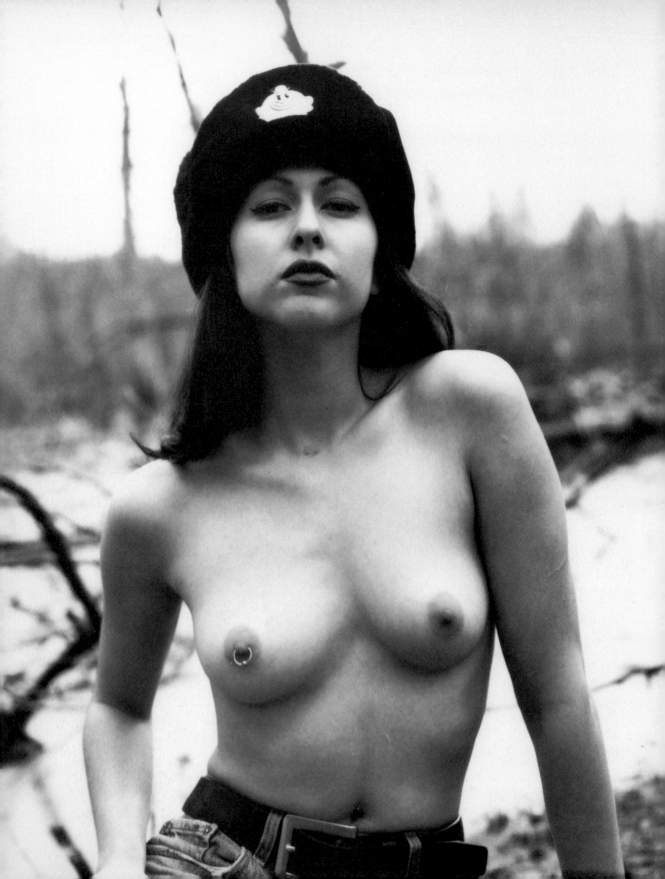

of the talking. They are angry: "If I was a mother, I'd try not to teach my children superficiality. I'd encourage them to get past modeling and be a person." Applause.

"These aren't people?" Dorothy is pissed. "And as if modeling is even an option to most people." She wishes somebody from *Playboy* PR was here to protect the girls and keep them from being made to look so…cheap.

"What did your dad think?" Montel asks Jennifer from Texas. Her hair is huge now and she's squeezed into a very small dress that barely covers her ass. Jennifer is pre-med. "My dad told me that there are people who say they're gonna do things and people who do them. He said I was a doer. He liked it."

"He liked it, huh?" Montel winks to the audience.

One lady says Marlee's mom is prostituting her daughter. Marlee holds back tears for the rest of the show.

Doni from Central Michigan is thin and has mostly straight hair in real life. On Montel's show, her poofy hair and sequined outfit make her look chubby.

LEFT: Amanda by C. Jason Moore

BELOW: Marlee by John Hall Photography, Phoenix, Arizona

A very angry college girl asks Doni, "Do you think college guys will, like, come up to you in bar for your mind after they see these pictures?"

"Anybody who came up to me in a bar didn't want me for my mind before these pictures." Doni has a heavy Midwestern accent that makes her sound like a den mother. Doni wants to be a schoolteacher, sex education. "Why can't a woman expose her body? Why can't a body be appreciated for what it is?" The audience is angry at these loose women.

Amanda takes off her sequined jacket during the commercial break, and a producer runs out and tells her to put it back on. She's afraid if she doesn't, *Montel* won't pay for her flight back to Georgia. Amanda has never done New York City before, let alone a national talk show. She puts the sequins back on but doesn't slip when she speaks: "This country has got to get over its hang-ups about the body.

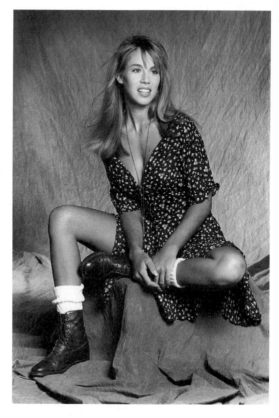

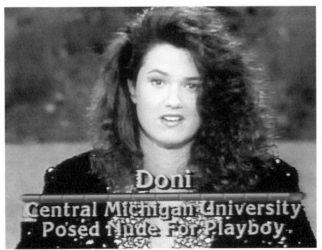

Doni
by Ken Siman

European *Vogue* has naked models all the time.... If you took our pictures from *Playboy* and put them in a woman's magazine, it would be considered very liberating," she says as the credits roll.

The show is over. Marlee bursts into the greenroom in tears. Her mother hugs her. "Have a cigarette, darling. You're going to have to learn to deal with bigots in life." The other girls come in a little later. They had to return their clothes.

"Did you see what they made us change into?" Jennifer asks.

"I felt like Liberace," says Doni.

"They were on a witch hunt, man," says Amanda.

Envy is inevitable on the beauty trip and I still remember the first time I witnessed it. I was in elementary school. My father had just come from work and made it a point to tell my mother that he'd seen a "real beauty" picking her nose at a stop light.

"You should have honked the horn and laughed in her face," my mother said.

There's a tingle of satisfaction that comes when those we envy are taken down. But even though these *Playboy* girls—except for Amanda—are the same types who snubbed me in high school, and even though I'm not into the *Playboy* look (I really do subscribe for the articles), I don't resent these girls for having their moments. In the same way a frustrated jock has done away with enough of his envy that he's able to scream in ecstasy during televised sports, I—a model wannabe—have enough admiration for beauty that it's easier for me to applaud than sneer at those who are able to flaunt it.

But if I'd been watching these girls when I was in high school or college, I probably would have fit right in with *Montel Williams*'s audience. It's not that I would have wanted to go to the same parties as these girls, it's just that it wasn't even an option. As my mother told me, "It's always nice to be invited, whether you want to go or not."

But the thing is, I am no longer in high school or college, and neither is most of the audience. We're ten and twenty years older than these girls. They are no longer our peers. We all go to different parties now. And we have a choice: we can celebrate youth and beauty, or—if it does not interest us—we can walk away from it. There's no need to play taunting games anymore.

"Put your coats on. We need to get you out now," says a frizzy-haired gum-popping producer around five feet tall. She has a heavy New York accent. "Come on, you have to leave now." Dorothy and I tell the girls we'll meet them in the lobby of their hotel and take them out to dinner.

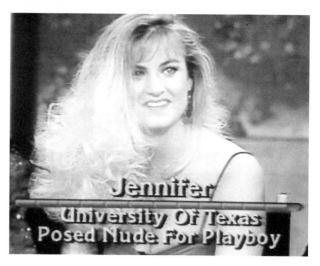

Jennifer
by Ken Siman

A modeling agent who checked the girls out at *Montel Williams* finds Jennifer sitting in the hotel lobby. "I know talent," he tells her. "I got the prettiest and sexiest girl in the business." His company is called Magnificent Models. He is in his sixties, rumpled black suit, white shirt, no tie, balding, big belly.

"Somebody gets a picture of my girls on his desk and boom. Action. I represented one young lady who was workin' in a pizza parlor. Now she's doin' the crème de la crème of the trade shows. Vanna White started with trade shows, you know. Do you wanna be part of the family? You're very pretty."

"That's real *nahce*," says Jennifer, holding a Magnificent Models brochure. "I'm real impressed. I'll call you when I'm back home."

"How about dinner?"

"No, thank you. I'm going out with the girls."

Mr. Magnificent Models whispers as he leaves, "If you don't want my brochures, throw them away. Don't pass them around."

Dorothy and I take the girls to a Spanish restaurant. The waiter wears a red dinner jacket and a black bow tie and has a heavy Spanish accent. The girls can't understand him so Dorothy explains the menu.

Dorothy had said how sometimes she get resentful of beautiful women, especially at parties and bars. Now she's in a restaurant with three *Playboy* models and she's being totally gracious. Maybe it's because there's nobody to compete for. There are no horny guys around, no model agents to give attention to the prettiest. All we can do is look at one another and talk.

We order the rice dishes, wine, and a couple whiskey sours. It's an hour after *Montel Williams* and the girls are still not over it.

"I am so pissed," says Doni.

Jennifer says she was surprised by the audience's anger. She never knew that people thought *Playboy* was so sexual.

"Seriously, y'all. I thought men used *Penthouse* for that," she says.

Playboy is not a magazine for aesthetes. And when *Playboy* does publish photos of women by Herb Ritts and Bruce Weber, work that's conceivably jerk-off material but still transcends the glossy-skinned spread shots, the subscribers complain. It's not what they want. They don't go for that black-and-white arty stuff.

It's obvious what the guys want to see, but what's in it for these college girls? They didn't get a lot of money, and none of them is looking for a career in modeling.

The girls will tell you straight out: They're proud of their bodies, and it's very gratifying to have the country admiring them. It means being accepted into one of the highest echelons of American beauty.

Sure, *Playboy* is mostly soft-core, but it's also pure Americana. And the photos are almost always of beauties in solitary repose—not couples. They never show "pink," or intercourse. It's so mainstream that Don Donovan (the man who drove Kelly and Amanda around Georgia) had his first grandchild pose with the girls. It's respectable enough that Jennifer can look me straight in the eye and say: "When I'm sixty, I can show this picture to my grandkids and say, 'See what Grandma did?'" It reminds me of what Bruce Weber said: There's a time when you're at the peak of your physical beauty and it's an incredible gift to be able to capture that moment and freeze it in something other than a memory.

Jennifer and Doni wince and say "Good Lord" when Amanda tells them where her body piercings are located.

"Doesn't that get in the way of sex?" they ask.

"No, sure doesn't," says Amanda.

"Amanda," they say, "you look so much more innocent in your photo than real life."

"I should have come with my pink parasol," she says.

"We were in a power position until that show," says Doni. "Back in Michigan today, the guys were so scared when they approached us for autographs." She thinks a mob mentality ruled on *Montel Williams,* that there was a lot of pent-up resentment of what women think they might be missing.

The girls are happy with their photos, all in color, but prefer the black-and-white arty ones that the subscribers trash. Doni and Jennifer don't think their bodies were airbrushed, but Amanda says they did embellish on her pubic hair.

Playboy does airbrush. Amanda remembers the issue—Sandra Bernhard was on the cover—when a girl's entire belly button was brushed off. "And sometimes the rugs don't match the drapes."

I tell everybody what a guy who works with Dorothy at *Playboy* once told me: Whenever guys find out where he works, they often say to him: "The girls are dumb and airbrushed, right?"

He said it makes them feel better to think the beauty that has power over them is dumb and fake or both. He tells them no, they're not dumb, just young. What would anybody sound like writing down their likes and dislikes at nineteen or twenty? And yes, they are airbrushed.

But why must they airbrush? A few girls are chosen—out of thousands of wannabes—for their beauty. Isn't that, plus good makeup and lighting, enough? It's not like they're aging film stars who need the touch-ups to keep their careers.

Dorothy says it's a look, and *Playboy* readers like it. The people hung up on airbrushing wouldn't read the magazine anyway. Dorothy's sister works in food advertising, and told her even hamburger buns are retouched before they are shown to the public. But that's the problem, the models can look too processed and synthetic, especially compared to the goddesses of fashion magazines.

Dorothy says *Playboy* readers are mostly suburban young white guys and they like their fantasy photos young, buxom, smooth, no edges, not even a pubic hair out of place, not even a wrinkle on the knuckles, and white. And this is what they are served.

Amanda, Jennifer, and Doni never have problems getting boyfriends. They go for cute boys but not beautiful ones because, they say, most of them are vain assholes and it's not worth the hassles. They say a guy has to be secure to go out with a beautiful woman, to deal with the attention she gets.

"I want a guy who'll always be willing to do things for me, always be full of surprises," says Jennifer. Female competition for guys is intense, especially in bars. "Girls are cats, y'all," says Jennifer. "Big time!"

"If I were dressed like I am now," says Doni, who's wearing jeans and a Western hat, "I'd get dirty looks from girls in a college bar. They stare. They whisper in front of you. Even on the *Montel Williams* show, I heard one of the girls in the audience say, 'Look at the bimbo.' When I'm confident and dressed up, the more nasty stares I get from women."

"Girls stereotype us, y'all," says Jennifer. "I had this roommate in college? And when she saw me for the first time, she ran out of the room and got real mad. Somebody had told her I was a Plain Jane, and when she found out I wasn't, she just freaked. She was so nasty to me. I swear, y'all, she made me cry every day."

But beautiful girls are nasty to each other, too, says Jennifer.

"One time I went to this bar in Dallas where a lot of blond girls go? There was a lot of competition. All these girls are staring at me in the worst way, like I'm a bitch for being there."

Doni isn't a blond Dallas girl, but a Midwestern bohemian. She says she just prefers not to wear clothes whenever possible. She may even go to a nudist camp this summer. "This is really me," she says. "What's the big deal?" Doni says the attitudes in Europe are so much healthier. Even homely people take off their clothes on the beach. "Nudity doesn't always mean sex. The point is to be free."

I am a frustrated exhibitionist and have always been envious of people who are unself-conscious about their bodies. But when it's hot outside and I see men walking the streets of New York shirtless, oblivious to their doughnut guts and hairy backs, my envy is mixed with an unforgiving sense of aesthetics. As a rule I think it's fine to walk around with no clothes on in your backyard or designated beach areas, but don't take off your shirt in nightclubs or on streets unless you are often mistaken for a Bruce Weber model.

Dorothy wants to know if the girls are given special privileges over people who are not good-looking. "I kind of feel guilty," says Doni. She first realized she was pretty in elementary school when a teacher told her she was going to break a lot of hearts. She wasn't sure if that was good or bad.

"It is easier to get a job," she says.

"It all depends on my look," says Amanda. "When I get pulled by a cop and I'm in combat boots, I get a ticket. If I'm in a dress he lets me go."

"When a cop pulls me over," says Jennifer, "and I get pulled all the time—I just smile and am happy. They go 'You're going eighty-five,' and I go, 'I'm always going eighty-five.' They just give me a warning. One time I was pulled over twice in ten minutes. I told the policeman, 'I just got pulled over ten minutes ago, let me go,'" He did.

Even though they were burned by *Montel Williams,* the girls are getting off being in New York City. "Let's go to a club, y'all," says Jennifer. Dorothy picks up the dinner tab, and the girls continue to talk about *Montel Williams.*

"If *Playboy* approached all those women in the audience who hated us and said, 'You're beautiful. You should pose for us,' all of them would be flattered and a good number of them would do it," says Amanda.

"It would be nice to be asked," says Dorothy.

10

dorothy

won't be posing in *Playboy*. Now she's more interested in getting *Playboy* to feature women who have more of an edge to them, a different look. She's made friends with one, Angeline.

*Maria Snyder
by Vangelis*

I go with Dorothy and Angeline to a party at Tiffany's for the model turned designer Maria Snyder. "She's a total enchantress," I tell Dorothy and Angeline. "I don't see how anyone could say no to her."

As soon as we walk into Tiffany's, a photographer hugs Angeline and tells her to pose with some other models. Angeline is tall and poreless and blond. She's in an orange dress with a slit in the bottom front. Her legs are long and shaved. She's paid the rent with modeling money for fourteen years.

"That's a cool way to be welcomed to a party," says Dorothy. We both slam back a glass of champagne while Angeline works the room. We can't find Maria Snyder. I think we've missed her.

Dorothy says that even though Angeline isn't the mall girl that most *Playboy* readers want (she's thirty-four, her breasts aren't huge, and she's styled in SoHo), it looks like she'll be able to get her in *Playboy*'s bisexual issue that's set to come out in a few months. It helps a lot that Angeline made a name for herself in the Big City with her same sex–safe sex poster by Steven Meisel. This is the first time Dorothy has had a crush on a *Playboy* model.

Dorothy thinks about beautiful lesbians a lot. Growing up, Dorothy thought she was doomed. "I was ugly and I was a lesbian and all lesbians were supposed to be ugly," Dorothy says. "I had no future."

But choosing not to pursue beauty got to be tedious for a lot of lesbians. Dorothy doesn't think lipstick lesbians are "appeasing the patriarchy" by having some beauty rituals similar to straight women. "Guys can look all they

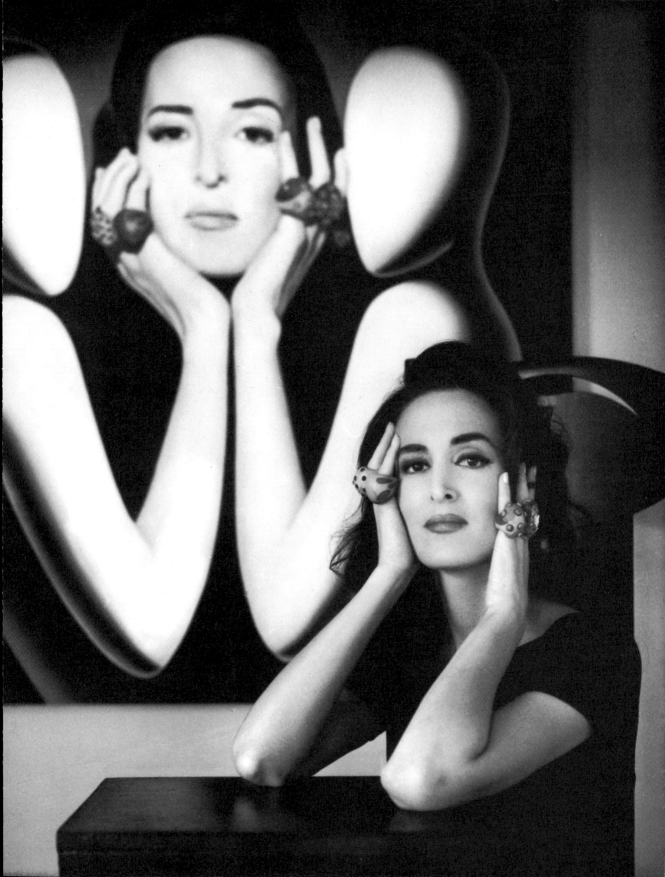

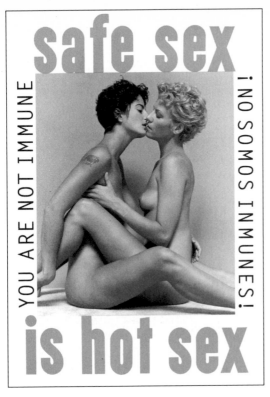

safe sex

is hot sex

YOU ARE NOT IMMUNE

¡NO SOMOS INMUNES!

ABOVE:
*SAFE SEX IS HOT SEX
photo by Steven Meisel,
courtesy of DIFFA*

RIGHT: *Angeline
by Rick Guidotti*

OVERLEAF: *Angeline
by Greta Olafsdottir and
Antoine Verglas,
courtesy of Angeline*

want, but they won't be able to get us," she says.

"Almost everyone I've met has a fantasy of being with a woman, and now it's okay for them to act on it," Dorothy says. "A lot of straight girls are willing to experiment because they see lesbians don't have to be ugly." The best thing about lesbians embracing beauty, Dorothy believes, is that "young dykes won't have to torture themselves the way I did."

We find Angeline and she leads us through the party.

I can't stand cocktail parties because I'm nervous to begin with and ran out of small talk a couple years ago, but going with a beautiful woman makes things a lot easier. "Let's have some fun," Angeline says. She taps people on the shoulder and looks away. She bums cigarettes and lights and gets them instantly, and dinner invitations, too. She even makes the fashion people who wear sunglasses indoors smile.

Angeline tells us it's hard for her to settle down with someone, even though she's thirty-four. For one thing, she's bisexual, and for another she's guaranteed new options every night she goes out.

Why settle for one person when an entire room is willing to be your suitor?

This is the power of beauty that Dorothy is preoccupied with. But power to what end? Having your speeding tickets fixed? Getting asked to dinner a lot? Better-looking dates? Smiles from strangers?

I always thought of power the way Roy Cohn did. It meant one phone call could take down an enemy or elevate a friend. And those who possessed it would usually not see beauty in their mirrors, but in the trophies of their power: the model on their arm, the pretty boy in their bed. In other words, the beautiful people have access to power, but rarely dispense it.

"The power of beauty is the power of the moment, the power of instant acceptance," says Dorothy. "But not getting that acceptance can put a chip on your shoulder that drives you to do extraordinary things."

"I think the beauty trip is more about pleasure than power," I say. "If you

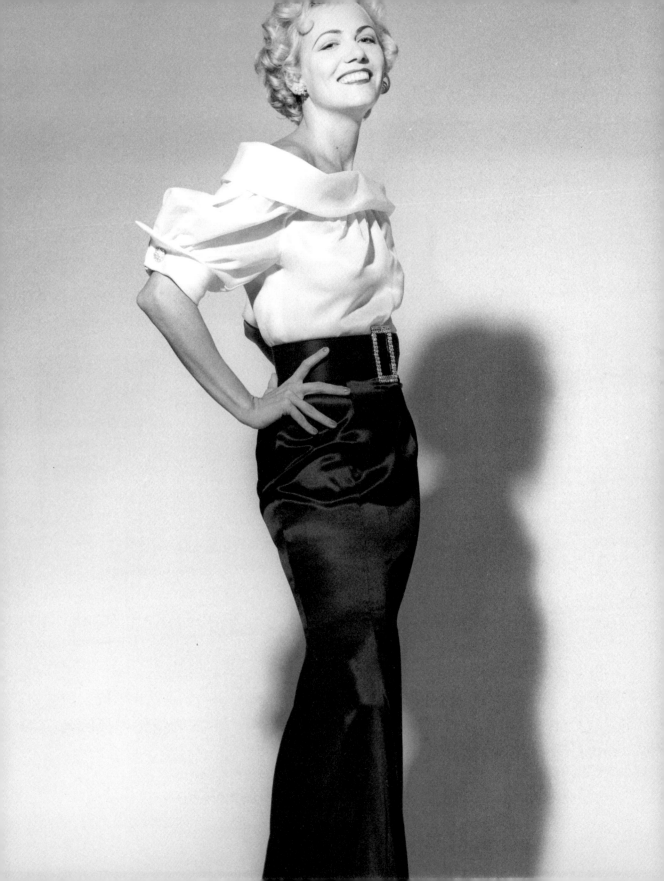

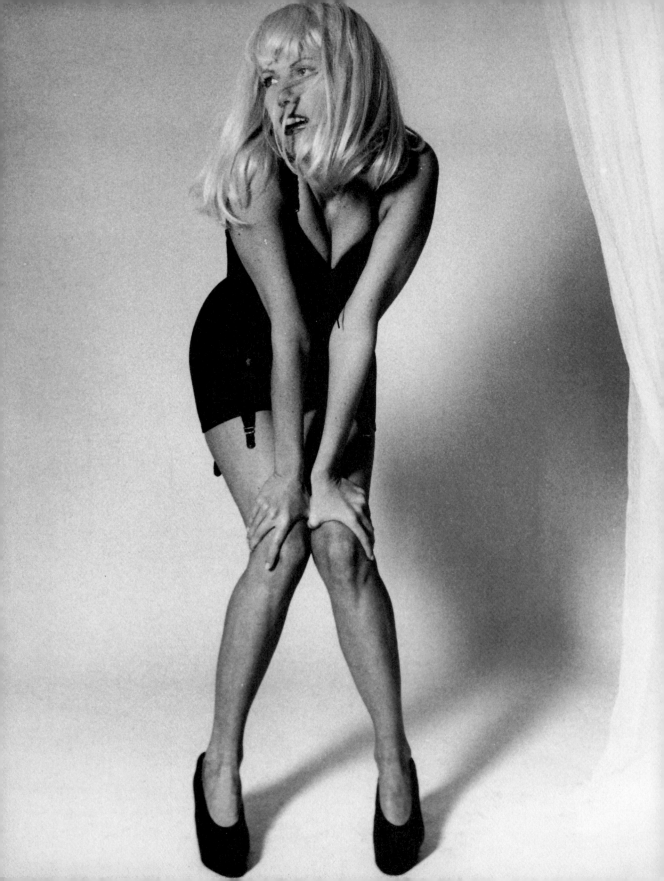

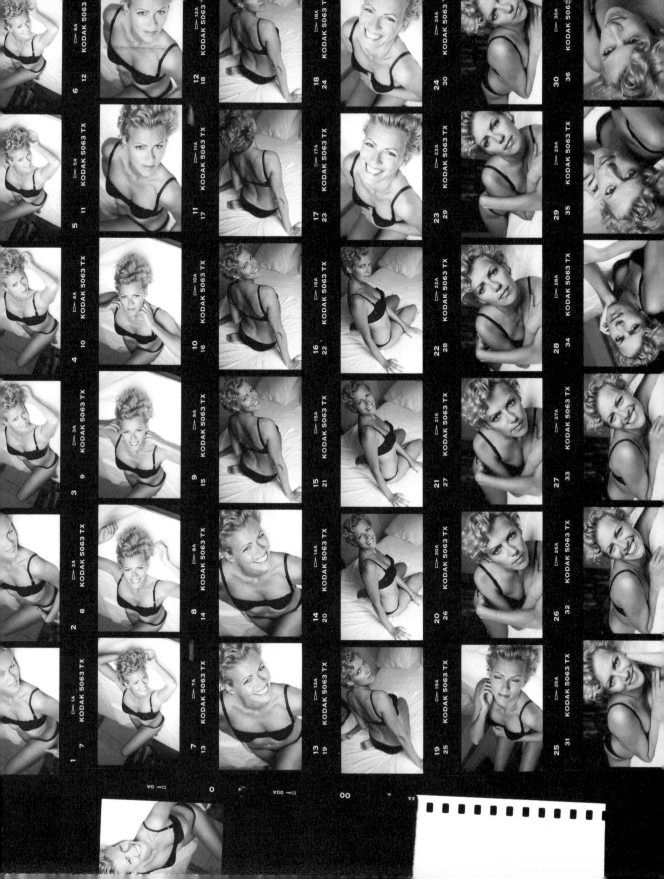

really admire beauty, then it's a pleasure just to look at it. It's not like we're trying to get authority over the beautiful people, or like they're trying to get authority over us." And since both Dorothy and I are attached, we haven't been trying to get laid. This makes it a lot easier for us to be bystanders.

Cocteau said, "The privileges of beauty are enormous." This makes sense. Beauty is more a privilege than a power. It's the privilege of getting paid to have your picture taken, of having strangers want to please you, of having access to fame and wealth. That might sound trivial, but it's not.

"Don't you think being adored and photogenic are two of life's pleasures?" I ask Dorothy. "Haven't we found that out?"

"Vicariously," Dorothy says.

11

a bunch of muscular Princeton boys are waiting outside McCosh Hall hours before the "Raising Women's Voices" seminar begins. They aren't here to check out the Women's Studies majors, but to see Cindy Crawford. She's going to be on a panel with Camille Paglia, Linda Wells, the editor-in-chief of *Allure*, and Alisa Bellettini, the producer of MTV's *House of Style*. They're all here to talk about the power of beauty. The panel, moderated by Cindy's sister-in-law (Richard Gere's sister) is sure to be packed, and the guys want to get front-row seats.

When Cindy walks in, the boys don't say, "Dude, I'd like to eat her for lunch." Their mouths just hang open and they applaud. Cindy Crawford is not a magazine-manufactured illusion. She is a cheerleader from DeKalb, Illinois, perfected for the world to fawn over: no baby fat, six inches of added height, and hair, makeup, and attitude that make her mysterious and wholesome at the same time. Her voice is not as riveting as her look, but it does not diminish the look because she never pretends to be untouchable.

Cindy, twenty-seven, says she came of age after the feminist revolution of the late sixties–early seventies and never had to prove she was as good as the boys.

Camille Paglia, MTV's Alisa Bellettini, Allure's Linda Wells, and Cindy Crawford at Princeton by Holly Marvin

It was a given, she says. She is now "president of a company that owns a product called Cindy Crawford." She knows the product won't sell forever, but now she makes millions and has her own show on MTV.

Cindy says she looks awful in the morning and doesn't like the fluorescent lighting in department store fitting rooms. I think she

83

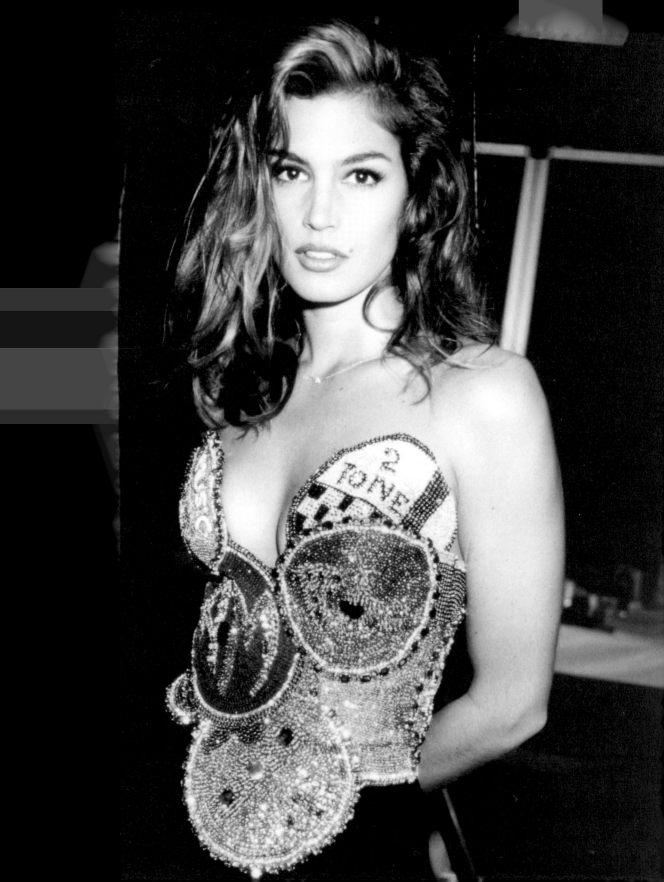

says this to comfort us; there are some complexions that glow even under fluorescence.

But a lot of the students are angry at her.

"Don't you cause eating disorders?"

Cindy is earnest: "Do you look at pictures of me and want to puke?"

"What about beauty that comes from within, why can't that be used to sell products?"

"It can't be photographed," says Cindy.

For the first time in my life, I side with the jocks over the nerds. The butch guys in front of me are getting a rise out of Cindy's presence; the academics are sullen and hostile. It's not that Cindy deserves an honorary degree, but as long as she's on campus, isn't the academy supposed to rejoice in the presence of youth and beauty instead of dismissing it as a corporate plot?

Then Camille Paglia says something that I'd never admitted to myself: "When I'm with a beautiful person, I [often] remember that for the rest of my life."

For me, that doesn't mean I slept with that beautiful person, or even had a conversation. It just means that sometimes a glimpse of beauty can be a moment that will never be forgotten, like seeing Christy Turlington in profile when she was having sparkles applied to her face, and watching a guy from my gym named Louis take off his shirt and show the most defined abs I'd ever seen. I barely spoke to the guy. I just handed him the phone number of Sean Kahlil, who photographs a lot of New York's muscle boys. The next time I saw Louis he was in a newspaper ad for a gym. I was so proud that I put that photo on the cover of my first novel.

What makes people angry—whether it's on *Montel Williams* or the Princeton campus—is that there's nothing fair about beauty. It didn't take training nine hours a day since the age of nine to become a star.

LEFT: *Cindy Crawford by Roxanne Lowit*

BELOW: *Louis by Sean Kahlil*

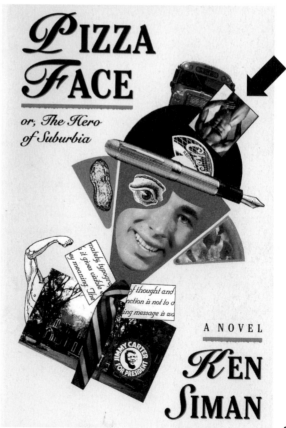

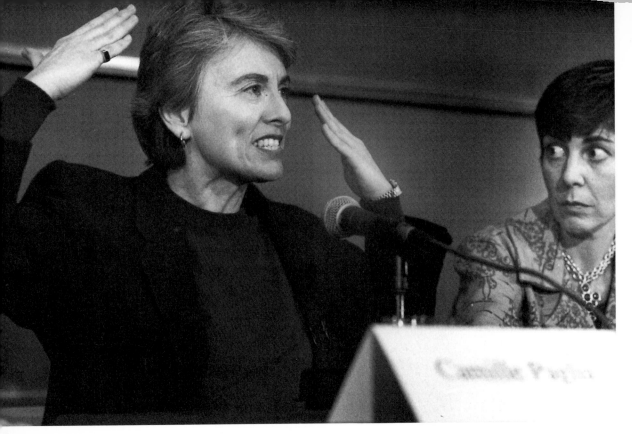

Camille Paglia and
MTV's Alisa Bellettini
at Princeton
by Holly Marvin

But hostility to greatness—even the most surface kind of greatness—breeds only denial and mediocrity.

It's like James Baldwin said: When little fish nibble at the body of a whale, that does not make them whales; the only result of that nibbling is "that there will be no grandeur anywhere, not even at the bottom of the sea."

But I did learn one thing at Princeton: It's impossible to have a dialogue about beauty today without discussing eating disorders, so I go to see Elly at the American Anorexia/Bulimia Association. And I remember how I hooked up with Elly in the first place. There was a segment about AABA on Cindy Crawford's MTV show.

12

i haven't seen Elly since the night we all went to Chippendale's and Scores. Since then, I've lost forty pounds because I've stopped eating fried flesh and dairy products. Plus, I do the StairMaster an hour every day.

Elly listens to some of my model stories.

"I have nothing against models," she says. "But they don't interest me. What makes me mad is when a lot of the people I work with [fighting eating disorders] are empowering the model, using her as the only powerful image of womanhood today. It is powerful, but in the end it's only a pretty toy used to sell products.

"By saying women's happiness and self-worth depend on what this sales toy looks like is dead wrong. We're making women out to be simpletons. There's a part of us, I guess, that can always be intimidated by beautiful people. But in the end, if you don't like what the model looks like, don't whine, just don't buy the product she's selling. Why do we cause ourselves so much pain?"

I guess beauty does not pain Elly because she hasn't experienced it as an extreme. She's never been spoiled as a beauty, mocked for homeliness, or ignored as plain. She says she's always been assured, though, of both her attractiveness and sex appeal.

But I get leery when Elly or anyone else says beauty does not interest them in the least. It's like money: some people are far more obsessed with it than others, but it's impossible to ignore.

"Elly, I lost forty pounds," I say.

"I didn't notice," she says. "When we talk I look into your eyes."

When Elly says things like this I want to shake her and say, "Elly, come on, you're human. You want a hunky boyfriend like the rest of us."

Elly says she's done that trip. She dated handsome jocks in high school and

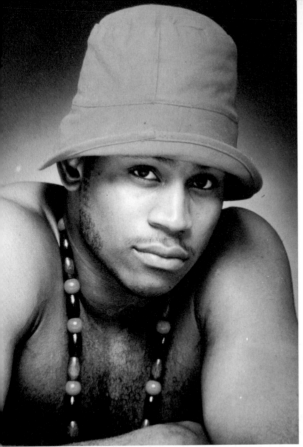

ABOVE: *L.L. Cool J*
by Ernie Paniccioli

RIGHT: *Jeremy Jordan*
by Ernie Paniccioli

once modeled in a shopping mall. She says she's over it.

"But what about the rest of us, Elly?" I ask. "We don't look to models for spiritual guidance, but wouldn't mind having a buff body."

"There's a healthy way of doing it," she says. She's going to talk to a junior high school class in Greenwich, Connecticut, and I come along.

Back in the seventies when I was in junior high, we were categorized by appearance: geek, prep, jock, cheerleader, redneck, plain, freak. Now there are students you can cram into these categories—except rednecks, because there aren't any in Greenwich—plus a lot more. There's sixties and seventies retro, hip-hop, pretty MTV boy...thanks to cable TV. The only shows on the idiot box I could learn style from were *Soul Train* and *The Hardy Boys*. And even the teen idols are buffer today.

Not long ago, teeny-bopper magazines would print nothing more intimate than the eye-color and fave toothpaste of the latest under-age male pop star. Now the same fanzines print full-color half-naked photos of young guys like L.L. Cool J and Marky Mark, along with their workout regimens. "I don't eat anything fried, marinated, or sautéed," said Jeremy Jordan in *Teen Dream*. (The caption underneath his photo read: "Jeremy shows off the benefits of his daily two-hour weight-lifting and running routine.") "You want to stay away from salt as much as possible.

That's what I did when I trained before my video, 'Wannagirl.' It's on MTV right now. I did a strict diet, and I got a Nutritionalysis at Gold's Gym. I was on that, and it really cut me down to eight percent body fat."

"I'd like all of you to tell me your name and a food that has a positive memory for you," Elly says to the Greenwich teenagers.

Most of their favorite foods are pizza, pie, and cake. One girl says watercress sandwiches. Now Elly shows them a Jenny Craig diet commercial. The people on the Jenny Craig plan are extra happy now that they've become slim 'n' trim!

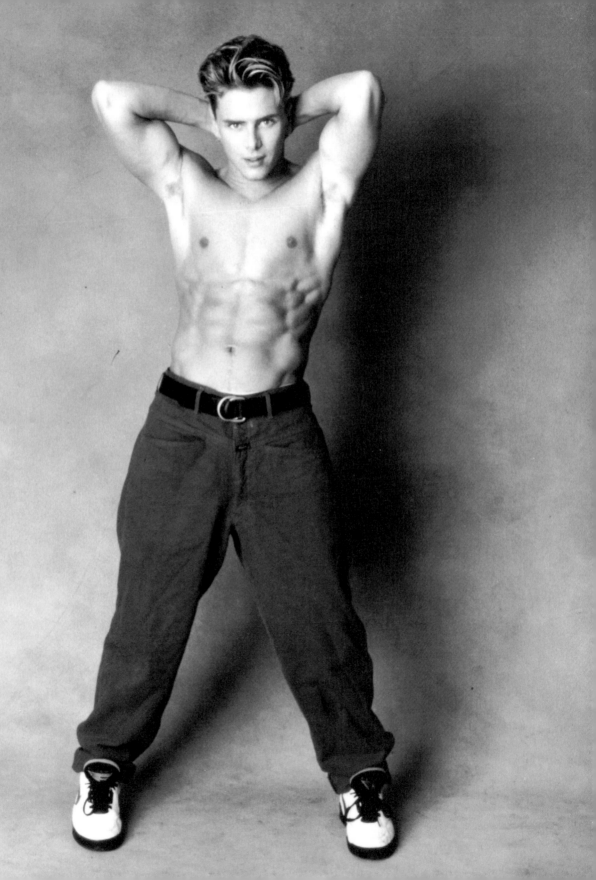

"You all told me that food makes you happy," Elly says. "But every day, you're confronted by a billion-dollar industry saying you'll become happy by not eating. [More important, Elly will say later, most of the teenagers' mothers are dieting, and the kids inherit the tradition.] This is a real conflict, right? How many of you have been on a diet?"

Almost all the girls raise their hands.

"Well, there's one thing that the diet industry isn't telling you: Diets don't work. Ninety percent of the people who go on diets gain the weight back."

She tells them about the Minnesota study. A group of men were forced to eat 1,570 calories a day (a typical American fad diet) for six months. The guys went nuts. Food was all they talked about, they became dispirited, reluctant to make decisions, self-centered and egocentric, and their quest for knowledge collapsed. It sounds like an American woman on diet pills.

If you insist on losing weight, Elly says, see a nutritionist and a doctor. Exercise several times a week. And eat healthy foods—vegetables, fruits, low-fat food—three meals a day. Never starve yourself; the process will make you dim-witted and irritating to be around, and you'll eventually gain back the weight. If you're serious about maintaining a certain weight, a diet becomes obsolete. Healthy eating is a lifestyle choice you'll have to stick with for the rest of your life.

"Most diets are examples of eating-disordered behavior," Elly says. "Eating-disordered behavior is much more common and not nearly severe as an eating disorder."

Most women have had eating-disordered behavior at one time or another. It's yo-yo dieting, obsessing on weight, having unhealthy eating habits. Elly thinks common sense and education can eliminate much of this. It becomes a rite of passage, a sign of womanhood, for girls to go on diets. Elly's hope is that diets will soon be like smoking and sun baking: Some will indulge, but they'll know the risks from the start. But unlike smoking and the sun—which provide imme-diate gratification—a diet is masochistic from the start.

An eating disorder can be one of several things: anorexia (starving), bulimia (bingeing and purging), and binge eating (uncontrolled eating). The National Institute of Mental Health says approximately 1 percent of adolescent girls develop anorexia and 2 to 3 percent of young women develop bulimia. Binge-eating disorder is found in about 2 percent of the general population—more often in women than men.

Eating disorders are incredibly complicated and not fully understood. The distinction between anorexia and bulimia wasn't made until 1979, and there's no conclusive verdict on what causes them, let alone cures them.

This much is known: Eating disorders often begin with intense dieting, another reason why Elly wants to take an ax to the diet industry. Why does the dieting become suicidal? Many agree that the cause is often some kind of familial or sexual conflict. The more the afflicted pay attention to how they look and what they put or don't put in their mouths, the less time they have to think about what caused them to be obsessive in the first place. "Eating disorders," says Elly, "are about pain and suffering and a cry for help. It's about having control over something when your inside is out of control." But some doctors think the cause is biochemical.

It's not certain how much eating disorders have increased over time. Elly thinks it's all about families and sex, and that it's more visible because we're allowed to talk about it, and more prevalent because neurotic eating is tolerated in our society. At the turn of the twentieth century, a woman suffering from inner anguish would maybe have fainted a lot instead of putting a finger down her throat.

So what do you say to a sixteen-year-old girl who sees a photo of Christy Turlington and thinks, "If I don't look like her, I'm a bad person"?

"When that happens," says Elly, "It shows what our society is lacking—a movement away from the home, away from civility and grace. And you can't blame that on the beauty industry. So many of the young women I talk to haven't learned basic coping skills. And that's the family's responsibility.... All I can do is hopefully educate a few people every day...."

Elly's got to get back to the office. Milton Bradley's come out with a bulimic toy called Eat at Ralph's. "To win," say the instructions, "stuff Ralph with all your snacks. But if he eats too much, it all comes back. Ages 5–up." Elly's got an appointment to talk with Milton Bradley's president. She'll set him straight.

I've got a dinner date with Carmen.

13

i'm in a French bistro between Fifth and Madison, waiting for Carmen. She has been a professional beauty since 1945. Her first *Vogue* cover was in 1947, and she's still in the magazines today, age sixty-two. Carmen goes by her first name, not to sound more like a model, but because her last name is so hard to spell and pronounce: Dell'Orefice.

Everyone in the bistro but me is in some kind of formal business wear and over forty. It's the kind of place that makes you wonder if the waiter is always this gruff or is it me? But then Carmen arrives and puts him in a good mood.

Carmen looks like a Botticelli painting—tall and slender with perfect posture. She has silver hair, almond-shaped eyes, and skin that has neither wrinkles nor marks. She's dressed casually elegant—a turtleneck, blazer, pants. Her speech mirrors her looks—deliberate but not forced.

Beauty is not always goodness, Carmen says. The face is not a mirror of morality. Some of the nastiest people she knows are beauties; some of the most noble are ugly. And what the camera reflects is confidence. A smarmy but self-assured businessman is more photogenic than a self-conscious philanthropist, for example.

No matter what she was going through, Carmen has always looked serene in photographs. This is how she supported herself and her family. "Beauty was my salvation," Carmen says.

When she was a kid in Manhattan, Carmen never dreamed of modeling. She always wanted to be a ballerina. Besides, her mother told her she had ears like sedan doors and feet like coffins. She always believed her mother. But the magazines loved Carmen and could make her look years older than thirteen. And she couldn't say no to the money. Ten dollars an hour meant seventy dollars a day

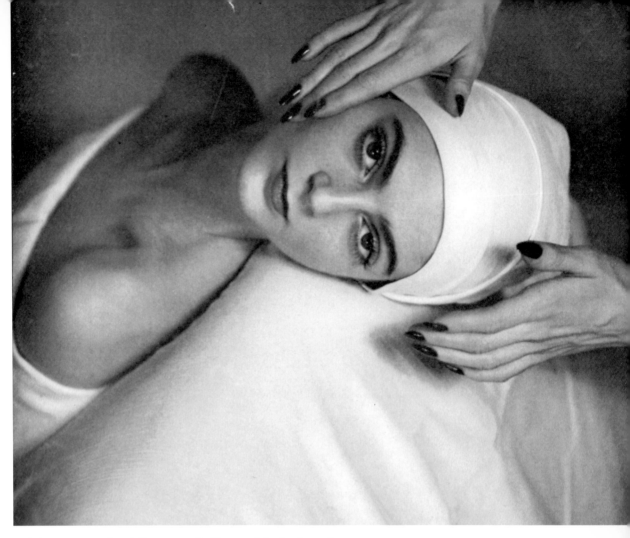

Carmen, face massage,
New York, 1946
by Horst

and the rent was thirty dollars a month. She was bringing home heavy money.

"I was at great odds as a thirteen-year-old with Cecil Beaton fawning over me in my braces and flat chest and oxford shoes. I was thinking, 'I have to get home to peel the potatoes before my mother gets home or she'll beat the hide off my ass.'"

For decades, Carmen was a star. She made the scene. Vreeland, Penn, Horst, Scavullo, Parkinson, and Avedon adored her. Joseph Kennedy tried to court her. As a young woman, she married twice but divorced both times.

"When men marry their fantasy, the relationship disintegrates when reality sets in," Carmen wrote in her autobiography.

Carmen tried a third time. She was in her forties and not working. Her husband thought her breasts could be a little firmer, so she went to see a cosmetic

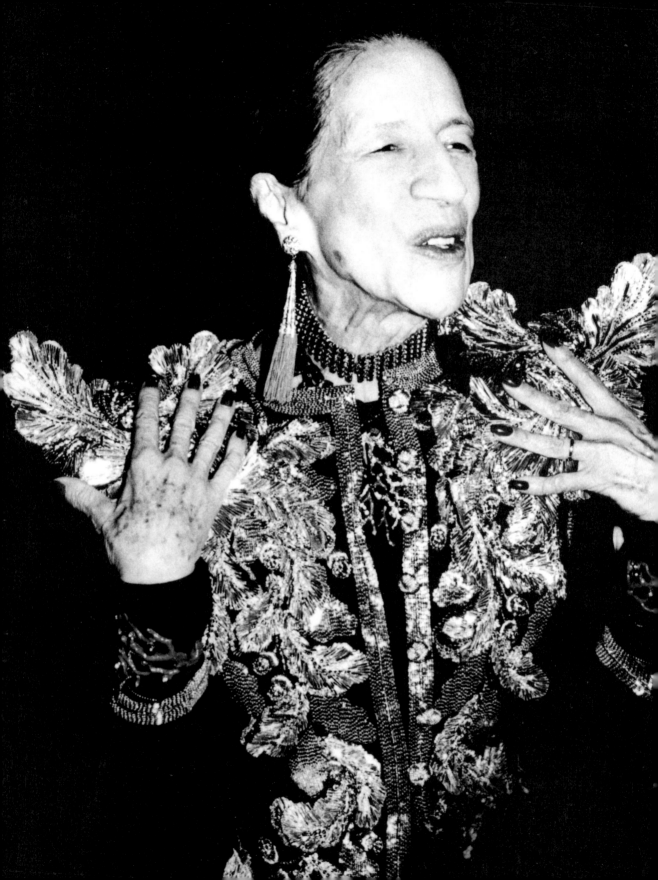

surgeon. He wouldn't touch her; she didn't need any work done.

One day Carmen's husband was in her face. She was expecting a kiss. Instead, he plucked a gray hair from her head and stared at it, horrified. He divorced her.

"I was a member of a generation of women who found their identities through men," Carmen wrote. "No woman whose youth and beauty brought fame and fortune terminates that period without fear."

Carmen was no longer modeling and no longer with a man. She thought maybe she deserved this downfall. She had exploited her appearance without bothering to develop much else. She was a basket case. What could she be? A secretary? A saleslady? A cleaning woman?

Carmen reminds me of Auntie Mame from the movies. Mame is the adored aristocrat who lost it all in the Depression and didn't have a man to fall back on. Mame tried to be a commoner; she was a telephone operator for a day and a saleslady at Macy's for a day and got fired both times. But Mame and Carmen are aristocrats in the best sense. They bring you up and make you feel like you're doing something right just to be in their presence. So instead of thinking, "Welcome to the real world, toots," you make a wish: A rich man will fall in love with them and bring them happiness. This is what happened to Mame and—in a way—what happened to Carmen. But the man did not give her wealth or a wedding, he just took her picture.

Norman Parkinson "came to my rescue like the knight on the white charger of my adolescent dreams." Carmen was forty-nine. The photos were fabulous, a big hit in French *Vogue*. Carmen has been working ever since. "There's only one thing I'm qualified for, one thing I have experience at, one thing I love doing."

Carmen says it took her years to accept how the world looks at her, and there's a degree of noblesse oblige that comes with the attention. "One learns the technique of being compassionately polite. You learn not to negate another person's feelings." In other words, if Carmen receives a compliment, she will not—no matter how she feels at the moment—say, "Are you blind?" She will say "Why, thank you," and often end with "sweetie," "honey," or "darling." Then there is the privilege of being a beautiful woman in a public place, which is the ability to control a moment without speaking.

Diana Vreeland
by Roxanne Lowit

OVERLEAF: *Carmen*
by Norman Parkinson at
ages seventeen and fifty-
seven, courtesy of Carmen

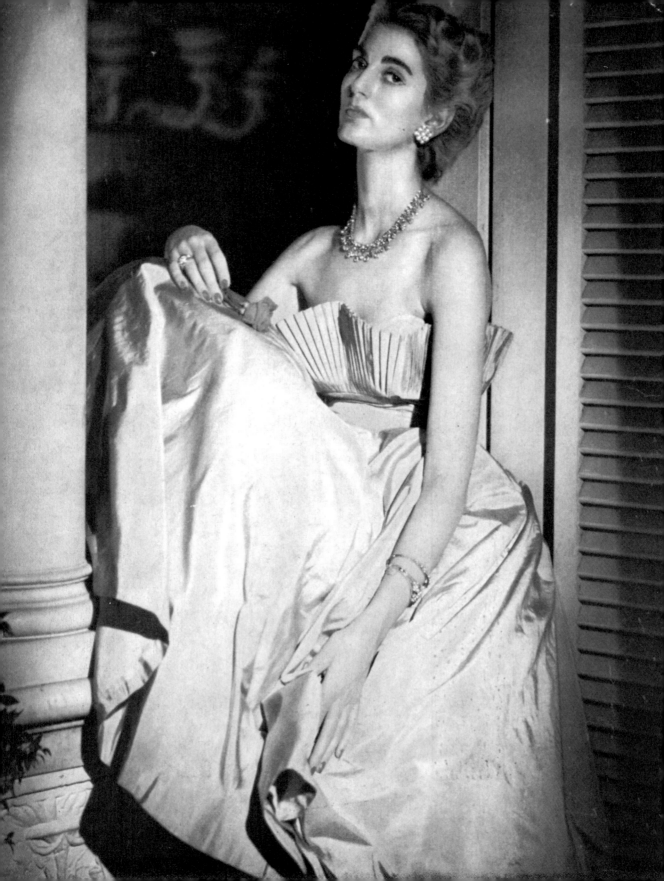

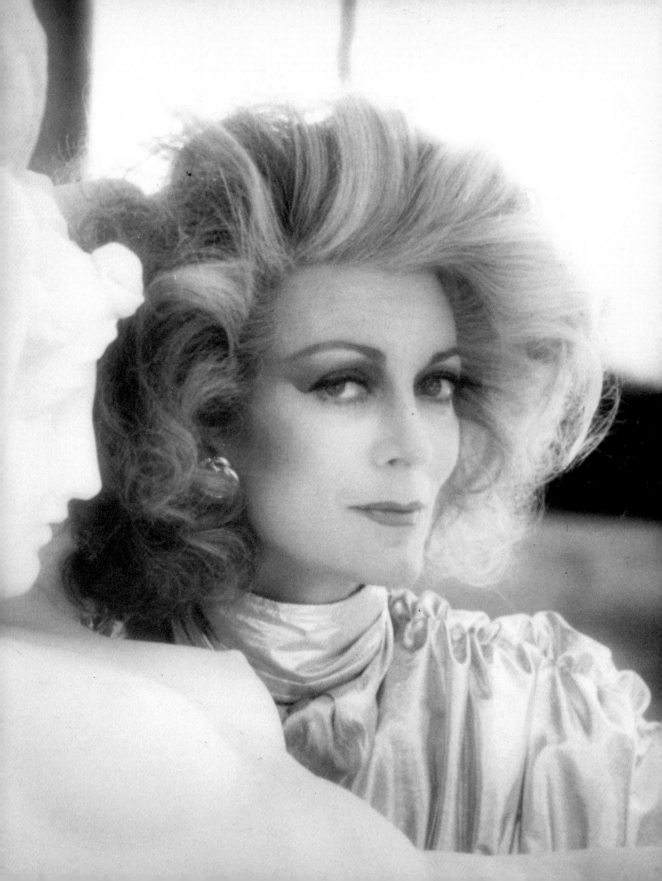

Carmen
by Frances McLaughlin-
Gill

"See that women over there?" Carmen asks. A fortyish woman who looks like a bank vice president sits alone at a table, frowning. "She looks so unhappy." Carmen smiles at her, the woman smiles back. "See how quickly that woman became infinitely more attractive?"

But, Carmen, I say, not everybody can smile and get that kind of reaction. If I smiled at that woman, she'd think I was trying to pick her up. If a woman who didn't belong in this joint smiled at her, she might think the smile was an insecure search for approval.

But who would rebuff the smile of a beautiful woman? Carmen says she can't "grandstand" like this everywhere. This is, after all, her turf: the Upper East Side. "I might not do this in a crowd of rowdies."

I don't even have to ask if Carmen's had cosmetic surgery. She'd already told *New York Newsday* about her silicone treatments. She's had sixty silicone treatments in her face, neck, and hands—two a year since 1962. "You're looking at a face full of silicone," she tells me.

Newsday's article was about the FDA's ban on silicone. Carmen defended silicone, said she never had a problem with the stuff. "All of New York is going to age overnight," she said. "All the movie people, all the theater people.... I feel really, enormously let down by this not being available."

Silicone wasn't used only for fake breasts. Since the 1950s, it's been called Cleopatra's Serum and was used to smooth out the faces of Eileen Ford, Calvin Klein, Helen Gurley Brown, and thousands of others, mostly rich people in New York and Los Angeles.

A couple of years ago, after I read in *Playboy* that Calvin Klein had silicone injections for his acne scars, I got a couple of treatments myself. The doctor took a needle and filled my flaws with little drops of silicone. Even an idiot knows that whenever you put a foreign substance into your body—whether it's acid, a metal plate in the head, or silicone—there's a risk that something can get seriously messed up. But unlike a metal plate, which keeps a brain in place, the only reason for silicone's existence is vanity. And I was vain enough to take the risks.

Dr. Norman Orentreich was society's—and Carmen's—silicone doctor. When Reagan was President, the doctor would fly by helicopter to the White House and treat the First Lady. That's why her face never wrinkled.

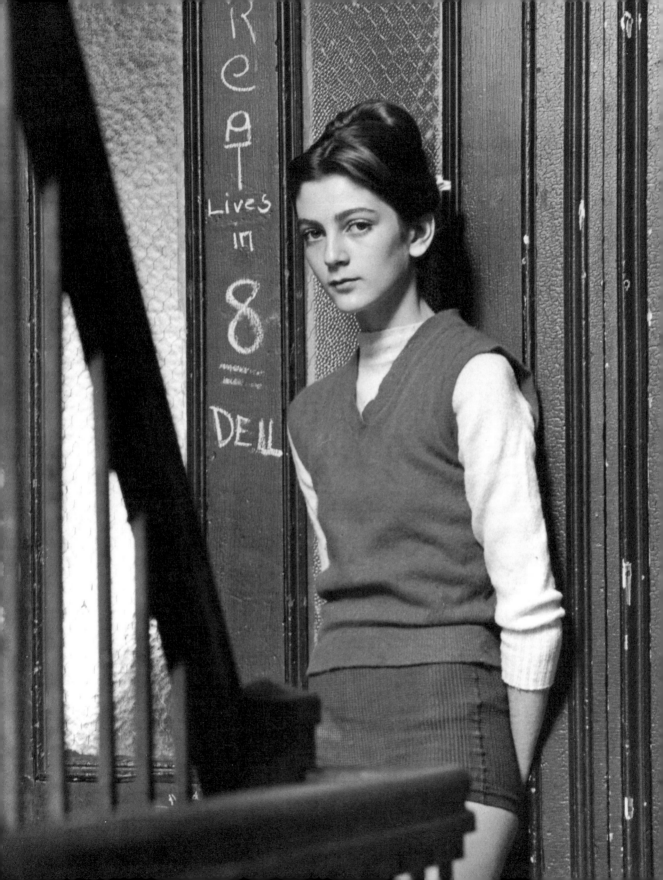

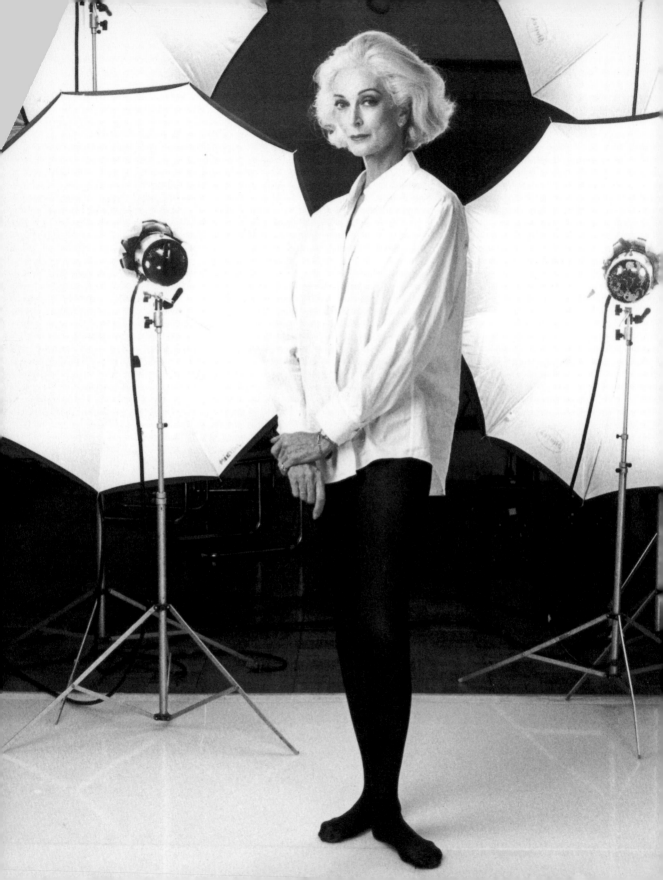

Most people's silicone stayed where it was supposed to. But when the silicone slid around, it destroyed some faces. It relocated, oozed, and caused bumps. So *60 Minutes* chased Dr. Orentreich down the streets of New York. He had no comment and was whisked away in a chauffeured car.

Carmen, I ask, didn't you see Dr. Orentreich on *60 Minutes?*

"They set him up," says Carmen. The women with mauled faces, she says, got impure silicone from a quack, some pure silicone from Orentreich, and when they lost their looks sued the wealthy one, Orentreich. I want to ask: Even if chances are that you (we) are 90 percent safe, isn't this a tame version of Russian roulette? And if the chamber is loaded, wouldn't this be a vain person's death? I do not ask Carmen these questions because I've already answered them for myself. What's really scary about silicone—any cosmetic surgery—is that if it slips, the vain person receives the ultimate punishment: a freakish face. This is why youth is beauty; it never has to be tampered with to shine.

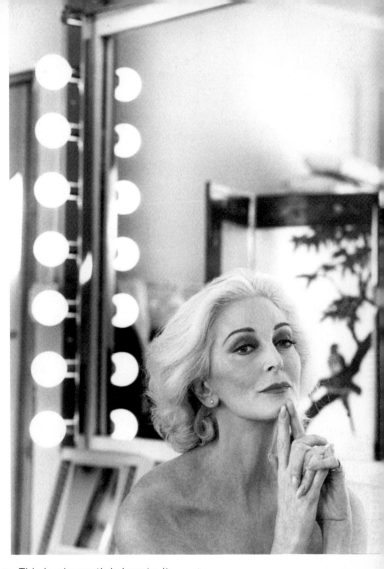

Carmen
by Michel Delsol

Be that as it may, Carmen says modeling has been the greatest lover in her life in the sense that she's been able to see the most wonderful places in the world with someone else's money. She's never had to work a nine-to-five job. She walks into a room and is guaranteed acceptance.

But Carmen never found her prince.

She's in *Worth* magazine this month because a financier took off with most of her savings. She's selling her silver now, her Parkinson prints, maybe, she thinks, her Park Avenue apartment. She's not in her teens or twenties, so even though she's still with Eileen Ford, she can't expect modeling money to flow.

She is not bitter, she says. This is just a challenge. She used to be a Catholic and still wears a crucifix around her neck, but her approach to life is more Zen. There is a reason for everything.

"I've transcended darkness through luck and fate.... I can't bring beauty down to physicality. I've devoted my life to living. Beauty is a flower, a fern that has lasted over a year. Maybe there's something in me that's beautiful because I've lasted so long. It's about balance in my life: the physical and the spiritual. Beauty is not disconnected from action. It's a moment."

Carmen and I eat dessert. The check comes and somehow Carmen had it taken care of. This is not how it's supposed to be. I protest.

"If you want to know what it's like to be a beautiful woman," Carmen says, "learn to accept things gracefully."

14

"**they do** look flawless," I say.

"Not a wrinkle on either of them. And they're both over sixty," says Dorothy.

Dorothy and I are watching a videotape of Barbara Walters interviewing Phyllis McGuire. Phyllis is the lead singer of the McGuire Sisters. They sang "Sugar Time," "Sincerely," and "May You Always" and were on the charts during the Eisenhower and Kennedy administrations. Dorothy and I are going to see them perform soon at a dinner theater in Illinois.

Barbara tells Phyllis she looks "dazzling" and asks her where she got the money to pay for her jewelry collection, which Barbara says is "bigger than Elizabeth Taylor's," and her Las Vegas mansion, which has a forty-foot-high replica of the Eiffel Tower indoors, a staff of twenty-eight, and security so tight that at the touch of a button steel doors hug the house.

Did you get it from Sam? Barbara asks.

Phyllis fell in love with Sam Giancana, the Mob boss best known for sharing Judith Exner with President Kennedy. Sam was the great love of Phyllis's life. He was gunned down in 1975.

Phyllis says she did not get her money from Sam. She had a lot of hit records and made wise investments in gas and oil.

Watching Barbara and Phyllis, I think: This is what plastic surgery is all about. Keeping people who have to face a camera for a living looking smooth. They get paid to be easy to look at.

But the eighties were for plastic surgery what the sixties were for sex and drugs. There is little subtlety left and it's available to everyone.

It used to be that people would whisper and wonder if Barbara Walters had had work done, and if so, where. Now, plastic-surgery articles in magazines list who

OVERLEAF LEFT:
*Phyllis McGuire
by Harry Langdon,
courtesy of Phyllis
McGuire*

OVERLEAF RIGHT:
*The McGuire Sisters
by James J. Kriegsmann,
courtesy of Phyllis
McGuire*

103

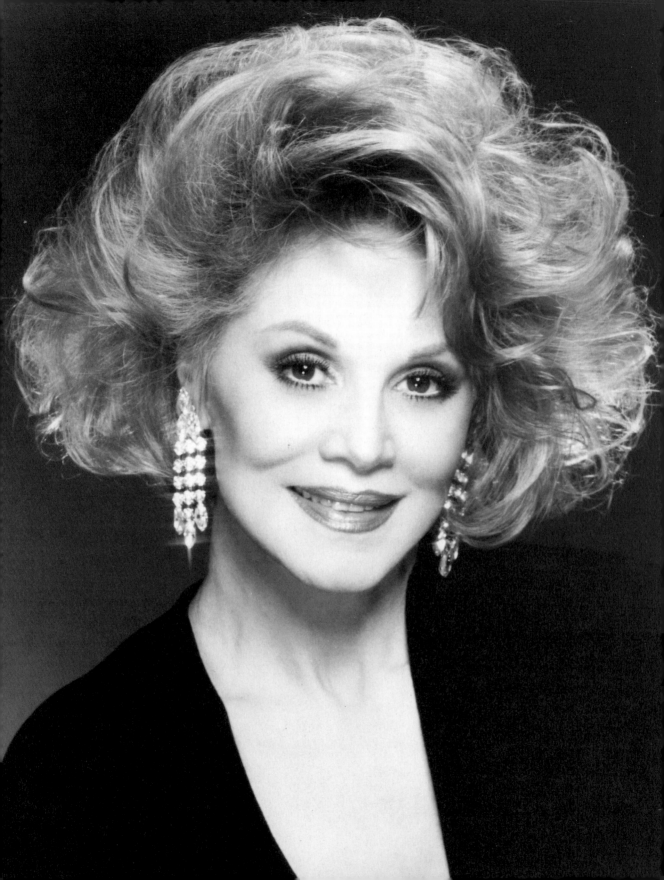

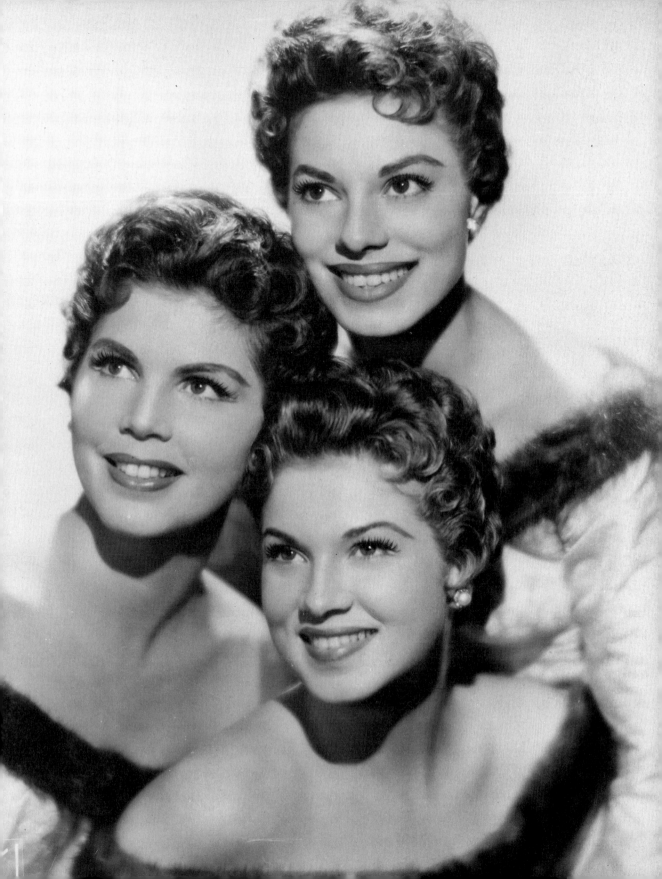

Lewis M. Feder, M.D.
beneath his portrait
by Michel Delsol

had what work done and who performed it. Want to know Barbara's skin man? Pick up the *Daily News* article on plastic surgeons to the stars: It's Dr. Michael Hogan.

I eject Barbara Walters's videotape and put in *Secrets of the Stars: A Fifth Avenue Doctor's Consultation on Cosmetic Surgery and Dermatology.*

"Oh, I know that guy," says Dorothy. "I've seen his pimple cream infomercials. He's a trip."

Dr. Feder talks about how to become more attractive. For Dr. Feder, looking more attractive usually involves having him suck fat from where you don't want it and putting it where you do. This is called liposculpture. He says a lot of the top models are asking him to take fat off their thighs and put it into their lips. Dr. Feder stores fat in his freezer. That way, when it starts to deteriorate, you'll always have your own supply waiting. Some plastic surgeons draw blood from patients, churn it into a custardlike gel, and inject it. But Dr. Feder says fat lasts longer than blood.

"Nature isn't always fair or kind," Dr. Feder says. "But there is a way of being reborn."

Dorothy and I listen to Dr. Feder talk about rebirth and wonder at what point we become flatout heathen on the beauty trip.

Or is cosmetic surgery the closest thing to a religious experience in this seemingly pagan world of beauty? It is hope. No matter how bad your appearance gets, you can always change. Here is a secular version of the Transfiguration, the glorified change in the appearance of Christ on the mountain (Matthew 17:1-9): "His face shone like the sun."

Who wouldn't mind having a Christ-like complexion?

I go to see Dr. Feder in person.

There's a huge portrait of Dr. Feder in his waiting room, next to the pay phone. It's of the "reborn" Dr. Feder. Since his first home video came out a few years ago, his hair has been lengthened and highlighted, and his cheeks are a lot bigger. Dr. Feder had some fat sucked out of his love handles and stuffed into his cheeks.

There's a sign on the receptionist's desk reminding patients not to miss Dr. Feder's TV show, *Here's Looking at You*—every Wednesday and Saturday night, channel 35.

"See how much better my skin is than yours?" Dr. Feder says to me. Dr.

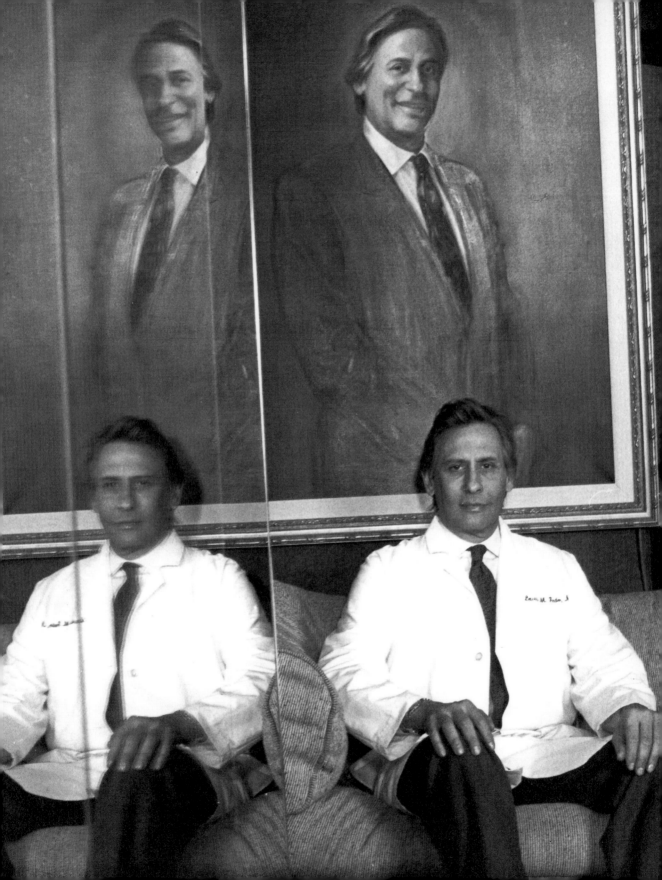

Feder is in his forties. He doesn't like to give his exact age; he jokes that he's eternal. He's not a kissable man, but he does have a great complexion. He says he peels his face weekly with chemicals.

Dr. Feder says I'm a good-lookin' guy, but he can make me a knockout. He says he can make me look like a movie star, but he doesn't say which one.

"Can you make me look like Billy Baldwin?" Really, all I want is perfect skin. But I was curious to hear what he'd say.

"First of all, I don't do noses. I would do liposculpture, eyelift, dermabrasion, maybe some cheek augmentation, lip augmentation...."

"Um, he has a lot of chest hair, too."

"I don't do that. People want it out, not in."

Dr. Feder wants to give me chemo-dermabrasion, a procedure he says he invented. He removes the skin on your face with a diamond wheel that rotates more than twenty thousand times a minute (your basic dermabrasion) and then takes off even more with carbolic acid.

I've already had two dermabrasions.

They did make me look better in the long run, but I'm not sure I want to experience the healing process again. My face was gone one week; it was just blood on a skull, like somebody poured red paint on my face. I wore an all-cotton goalie mask on the ride home from the doctor's so I didn't frighten motorists. Then my face became a scab. I could leave home without upsetting people after two weeks, but I looked like a reddish skinless grape for months.

"I'll think about it," I say.

Some people have dermabrasions to remove wrinkles.

Dr. Feder says a wrinkle is a deformity because "it is away from the accepted norm of society and makes people feel uncomfortable." In other words, everybody will have a deformed face at some point and will need Dr. Feder's help to be redeemed.

I let Dr. Feder give my face a light chemical peel, but am required to pay for it beforehand. Dr. Feder rubs an acid-laced Q-Tip on my face and asks me where I went to school. I'm never good at small talk, but it's even harder when having acid applied to my face. Suppose he brings up politics or religion and I say the wrong thing?

"UNC–Chapel Hill."

"Lots of beautiful women there, I bet," he says. "I love beautiful women. If there's a party with beautiful girls, I'll be there."

I want to say, "Get real, girlfriend, would a straight guy go through what I'm doing here?" but I feel the acid tingle on my skin.

"You got that right, doctor," I say. "Lots of babes."

I walk out onto Fifth Avenue. The peel made my face red, so I'm too self-conscious to go on the subway. I get a cab. The guy's playing disco from the Middle East loud enough that I can talk to myself without him noticing.

Why am I, a six-foot-five, two-hundred-pound man, looking to Barbara Walters as a skin role model instead of Tommy Lee Jones? Tommy Lee Jones has sorry skin, but he's so cool and tough in the movies that they call it rugged, a face that shows he's lived. What's wrong with a face that shows you've lived?

I try to answer for all of us—the wrinkled, the sun damaged, the acne scarred, the self-conscious, the vain. We want our experiences to show in our eyes, our walk, our speech, our manner—but not our complexion. Beauty is pure, not porous.

While I decide whether or not to let Dr. Feder work on my face so I can "look like a movie star," I remember one of his beauty tips: "Try to make your face not react to every emotion. You strain the muscles, causing more wrinkles. If you frequently respond with very great emotion, try to cut back. [If you wish to practice] sit in front of the mirror and talk to yourself. Try not to respond to every thought with a facial grimace. Get on the telephone and talk in front of the mirror and [never] make a big frown line."

Maybe I should get a second opinion.

My mother always told me, "If you have to find a good specialist, find out who your own doctor goes to." She was taking about podiatrists, not plastic surgeons, but she was right.

I don't have a regular doctor, only a dermatologist, Dr. Mary Ellen Brademas. She is one of the few people on the trip who is happy to talk about beauty *and* blood. Most aesthetes do everything they can to avoid ugliness. Dr. Brademas will wear Chanel while needlepointing seat covers inspired by eleventh-century drawings of a proctologist removing hemorrhoids.

"See the blood coming down?" she once said to *Allure* magazine. "And this is

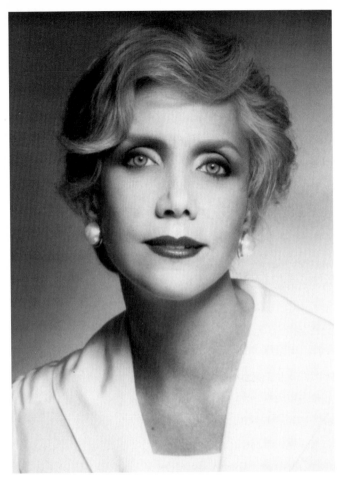

*Dr. Mary Ellen
Brademas
by Gary Ryan*

a retractor to spread apart the buttocks. I love to do needlepoint."

Dr. Brademas put me on Accutane for five months. That was over a year ago and I haven't broken out since.

Dr. Brademas says she hasn't seen Dr. Feder's TV commercial, and that I shouldn't be trying to look pretty; there's nothing wrong with the way I look now. But since I'm obsessed, she says I should see Dr. J. G. McCarthy.

"He did me," she says.

I thought Dr. Brademas was forty, but she didn't even go to med school until she was thirty-eight. Before that, she was a model in Michigan. She's fifty-five now, old enough to be my mother.

"See," she says, pointing to a scar under her chin. "I had a tuck." She also had the bags under her eyes removed.

Dr. McCarthy's office is on Park Avenue, a five-minute walk from Dr. Feder's. I'm in the waiting room with a teenaged girl and her mother. They might be trying to figure out what my flaws are, so I pick up a *Harper's Bazaar* and put my head down. I figure the girl is as self-conscious as I am, so I don't look at her. But I take a quick glance when it's her turn to see the doctor. She looks fine to me.

Dr. McCarthy meets with me in a dimly lit, classically–styled drawing room. He asks what I've had done and what I want done.

"If I have another dermabrasion will I have perfect skin?"

He takes me into his fluorescent examining room, then back to his office.

"Everybody wants good skin. I don't care who you are," he says. "The skin on your face is the way you present yourself to the world.

"But when it comes to facial treatment, you have to keep your feet on the ground, you have to be practical. First you have to be convinced that what you'll be doing isn't harming you. And you should never undergo anything unless there's going to be significant improvement. The deeper you go with dermabrasion, the harder it is to heal yourself. So having a third would produce few benefits with some risk. I wouldn't recommend it," he says.

I'm sort of relieved, though I'd been hoping all along that somebody could manufacture some perfect skin for me. At least now I know it's not possible.

When people talk about plastic surgery, they often talk about Michael Jackson having his race erased and Cher having her ribs removed.

There are extremes in everything, but this is not what plastic surgery is about.

At its best, plastic surgery can make celebrities more photogenic. It can get rid of a sagging face, a double chin, the bump on an insecure teenager's nose.

Dr. McCarthy says he changes fate only when he corrects severe deformities. "When a child has a birth defect, I try to have that child looking better by age four—before the child starts school and is treated differently by his or her peers."

Dr. McCarthy comes from a Massachusetts family, and seems almost Puritanlike. His mother was in her eighties when she told him that she wished she'd had a face lift. "I almost fell over when I heard that," he says. Plastic surgery isn't decadent, he says. It's just that everybody is allowed to talk openly about it now. The search for youth and beauty is eternal, he says. Look at Ponce de León and the Fountain of Youth. The only bad thing about plastic surgery's popularity, Dr. McCarthy says, is that there are a lot more quacks these days.

"There's a great quote I must find for you," Dr. McCarthy says. He stands on a ladder and pulls a book from the shelves. "Gasparo Tagliacozzi, the sixteenth-century founder of plastic surgery, said: 'We restore, repair, and make whole parts...which nature has given but fortune has taken away, not so much that they may delight the eye but that they may buoy the spirit and help the mind of the afflicted.'"

So plastic surgery cannot manufacture beauty, but it can make people less likely to chastise themselves when they look in a mirror, less likely to be a wallflower at a social function. It changes fate only when a deformed person is made normal-looking, or when a normal-looking person trying to be prettier gets botched.

But plastic surgery makes it almost impossible to end the beauty trip. For

though it can't create perfect skin, it can (with numerous follow-up appoint-
ments) keep a face virtually wrinkle–free.

So plastic surgery's popularity will continue to grow unless we decide that
wrinkles look better than pulls, or when—like silicone—the benefits aren't worth
the risks, or when—like cocaine—it becomes a symbol of having too much time
and money.

15

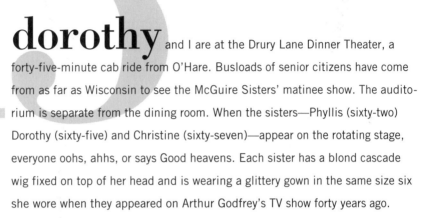

dorothy and I are at the Drury Lane Dinner Theater, a forty-five-minute cab ride from O'Hare. Busloads of senior citizens have come from as far as Wisconsin to see the McGuire Sisters' matinee show. The auditorium is separate from the dining room. When the sisters—Phyllis (sixty-two) Dorothy (sixty-five) and Christine (sixty-seven)—appear on the rotating stage, everyone oohs, ahhs, or says Good heavens. Each sister has a blond cascade wig fixed on top of her head and is wearing a glittery gown in the same size six she wore when they appeared on Arthur Godfrey's TV show forty years ago.

If you were sitting in the front row and brought binoculars, you could see that the McGuire Sisters are attractive women in their fifties or sixties. But nobody brought binoculars. And as Dorothy and I watch the audience—smiling, nodding, holding hands if married—we try to see the sisters the same way they do:

"Good lord, they haven't aged a year!"

"And *Christine* is a great-grandmother!"

"They're beautiful!"

And they don't need to lip-synch. They sound the same live as they did on my mother's hi-fi.

Fred Anthony stands in the back of the auditorium, next to the lighting booth. Fred is the man who styles the sisters and makes sure they are always singing in a flattering light. Fred believes in beauty for beauty's sake. His job is to style Phyllis and her boyfriend, and travel with the sisters when they tour.

Dorothy and I make our way over to Fred after the

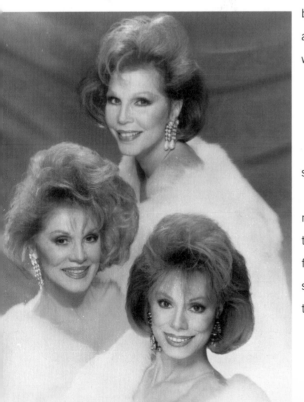

The McGuire Sisters by Harry Langdon, courtesy of Phyllis McGuire

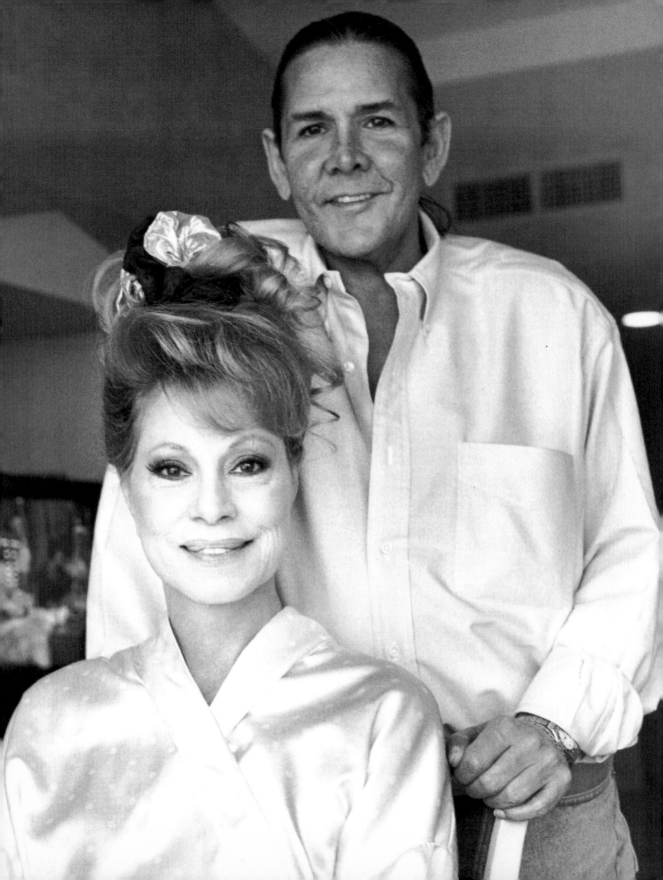

show. It's still afternoon, so dinner is not served with this performance. But the audience is satisfied: they can't get over how good the sisters look and sound.

Dorothy McGuire and Fred by Michel Delsol

Fred's forty-five years old. He has shoulder-length hair, and sometimes strangers call him ma'am. Fred invites Dorothy and me into the residential area of the dinner theater where the owners live. Everything is clean and carpeted. Phyllis is talking to the owner's wife. Barbara Walters was right: Phyllis looks great up close.

I remember what Billy Beyond told me about older stars who've had work done looking scary in the real world, but the only thing I'm scared of is being improper. I have so many questions for Phyllis, but Fred tells me only Barbara Walters can get away with asking them.

"Did Phyllis see Oliver Stone's movie about JFK's assassination?"

"I don't know," says Fred.

But evidently Phyllis told Fred that it was okay for Dorothy and me to ask him about her beauty rituals.

Fred says he "stopped dead in his tracks" when he first saw the McGuire Sisters. He was a pretty five-year-old boy in Miami and already knew he was going to be a celebrity hairdresser. He was holding his mother's hand as he crossed the street.

"Mommy, Mommy," he said. "Look how beautiful!"

Phyllis, Christine, and Dorothy were all dressed in navy blue. They were getting out of a navy blue limousine, the door held open for them by a black chauffeur in navy blue.

"I was always fascinated by anything that made people look beautiful," says Fred. "There was a lady from my neighborhood that went to Switzerland [for plastic surgery] every year and came back each time looking younger and more fabulous."

The neighbors would come to Fred's bedroom to get their hair done, but his parents didn't like all the traffic in and out of the house. So a neighbor lady sponsored him in her garage. They'd sit in patio dining chairs while Fred worked. He was so good that nobody ever complained about the car fumes.

Fred kept cutting hair. His face broke out bad and he wasn't as pretty as he used to be. He wanted to look like his mother, not his father. He started getting work done. His forehead was widened with a piece of latex foam placed under the skin. This also smoothed out the forehead veins. He's got silicone cheek-bones. He wanted a cleft in his chin and did it himself with silicone, cortisone, and a toothpick.

By the time he was doing celebrities in New York City, Fred would wear a wig on the days he wanted to be called Felicia. He took birth control pills because the estrogen gave his pecs a soft bosom effect, but he never had his manhood worked on.

"You know, Fred, Dr. Feder will put fat in your penis if you ask him."

"That's nothing new," says Fred. A few of his friends had silicone put in their penises to make them more lumberjack-like. One guy overdid it and died.

Fred's got the dish on everything. He says he touches women so much they instinctively want to reveal themselves to him and get rid of what's bothering them. Phyllis calls it "girlfriend time" when she and Fred dish.

Dondi,* "a prominent Chicago businesswoman specializing in entertain-ment," and her assistant, Rollo*—both friends of the dinner theater owners—are now talking about the work they've had done. Dondi is blond and over forty but looks my age. She gets Fred to promise that before he leaves he'll do her hair and share some of his glycolic acids. They're for facial peels, Fred says. Prescription-strength.

Dondi and Rollo, who is thirty, say they love to get silicone injected into their faces. It keeps Dondi young-looking. And Rollo was in a nasty car wreck but now you can't tell.

"It's illegal now," I say.

Yeah, but there's a mercenary that makes the rounds.

"You trust her?"

"Of course," Dondi says, and Rollo nods. It's the American Medical Association that got silicone banned, they say. The AMA hates silicone because it kept people from getting more expensive face lifts. It's all about money, they say. They're not worried about their faces exploding.

Fred's going to do Dondi's hair now, so Dorothy and I will meet him at the hotel for dinner.

*Not their real names.

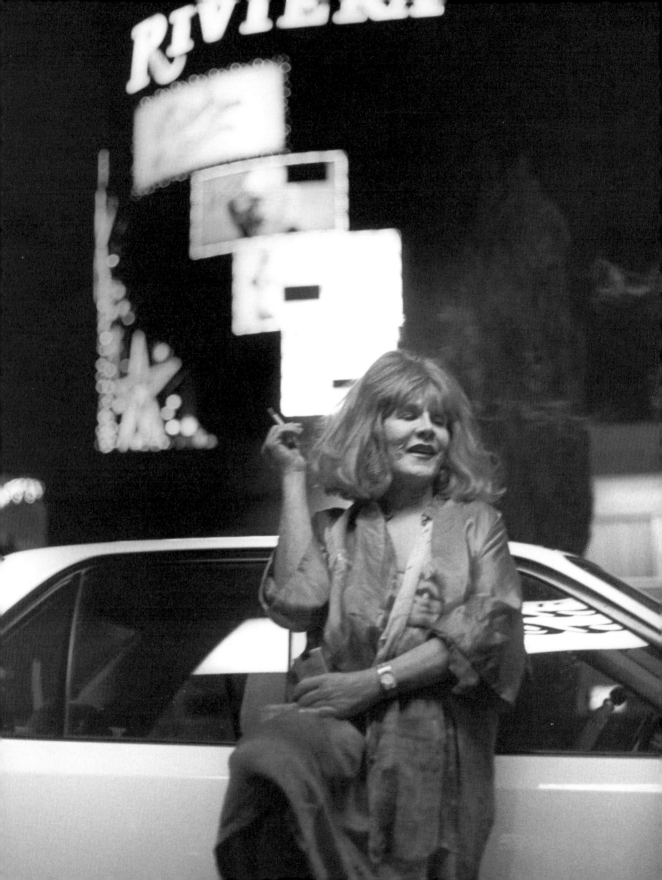

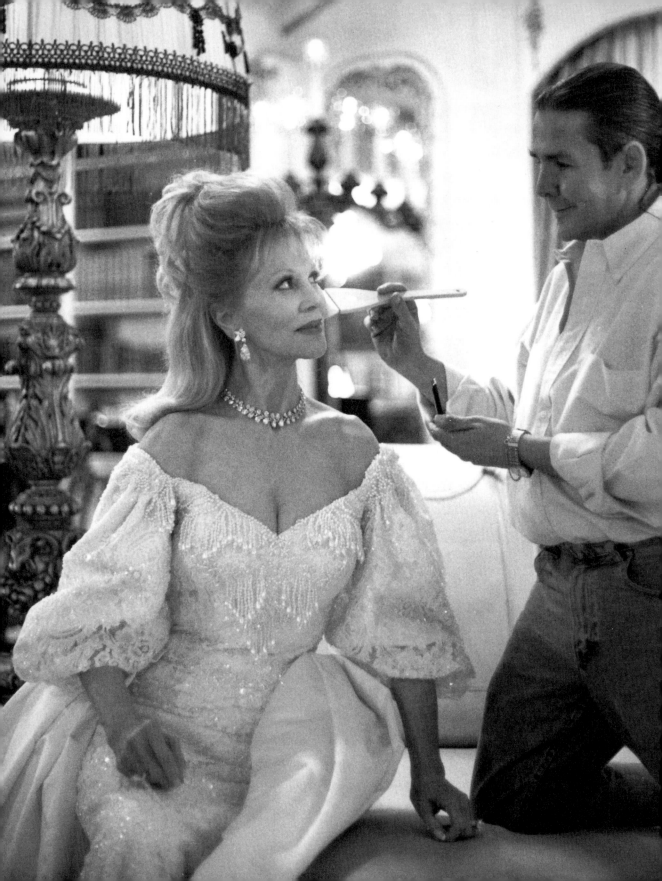

"So, Dorothy," I say. "Would that audience today have been as excited if the sisters had never seen a plastic surgeon? Isn't show biz about fantasy?"

"Yeah," says Dorothy. "But when do they stop? When do they allow themselves a few wrinkles?"

But it's a question of aesthetics, not ethics, I say. "Do you prefer the no-wrinkles look or the totally natural look? And we shouldn't answer that until we get wrinkles ourselves."

*Phyllis McGuire
and Fred
by Michel Delsol*

Fred orders a rusty nail with his steak.

"Tell us how you hooked up with Phyllis," Dorothy asks.

It was Christmas week in 1981 at the Dinmar Salon on Madison Avenue; the place was packed.

Margaret, the owner, said to Fred: "Dahling, do me a favor. Take care of Ms. McGuire."

It didn't register that Ms. McGuire was *the* Ms. McGuire, one of the women in navy blue.

Fred said, "Margaret, please, I've got Margaux Hemingway coming."

"You know how to charm these lionesses," Margaret said.

"So I started to do this woman. I thought she looked like Faye Dunaway. She had on dark glasses, a mink hat and coat, and had cheekbones to die for. But her hairstyle was old and the color was bad and I told her so."

"Well, what would you do if you could do anything you wanted?" Ms. McGuire said.

"With that I took a spray bottle and sprayed her hair down and cut it and bobbed it and threw a rinse on it. It wasn't until I had blown her hair out that I knew who she was."

Phyllis loved Fred's do. She sent a limousine to get him on New Year's Eve so he could brush her out in her apartment. When he got back that night, there was an "incredible Oriental flower arrangement and four bottles of Cristal."

Phyllis was moving to Vegas and asked Fred to write down all of his needs, everything he wanted in a salon.

"I hadn't planned on coming to Vegas," Fred told Phyllis.

"Oh, you will," said Phyllis.

"She knew where I breathed," says Fred. "She seduced me and treated me like a star."

So when Fred needed to leave New York to clean himself up, he had a job waiting in Vegas and has been there since. He lives in a hotel and can see the lights of the strip outside his window.

Fred doesn't work in a salon now, not even part-time. Phyllis and her boyfriend get all his attention. Fred travels a lot. He attends to the sisters when they tour and takes care of Phyllis's boyfriend—a prominent Las Vegas casino owner—when he goes on business trips. The guy is such a whiz at business that he doesn't have the time or inclination to color coordinate, so Fred picks out his outfit the night before, and makes sure it's laid out and pressed for the morning. Fred also provides him with plastic surgery tips.

Dorothy says she comes from a family that thinks plastic surgery is ethically wrong. "It's definitely a superiority attitude," she says. "The same kind that says beauty is not something to be discussed."

"Yeah," says Fred. "My mom had that attitude, but she had perfect skin, too."

Fred's into transfiguration. "Whenever I can portray inner beauty on the out-side, I do. The most gratifying experience for me in New York wasn't doing the celebrities. "Once," he says, "a girl from Ohio came to the salon, a temp from IBM. She didn't know what mascara was, she only wore lip gloss. She had very unappealing permed hair. But she had the most incredible bones, the most beautiful skin. I figured if someone saved up their money to come to me, they deserved the same treatment I'd give a star."

But the girl couldn't come back when she found out what the star treatment cost. Fred told her not to worry; one day she'd be able to pay him back. Fred worked on her free of charge for almost two years.

"And sure enough," says Fred, "one day she came to me with a blank check. I burned it. We called for champagne and caviar and celebrated in a little gar-den outside the salon. She went from being a Plain Jane to a beauty, and from a temp to a bigwig at IBM. And each time she hired somebody new, she'd send them to me on their first day."

Fred has another rusty nail. He pats his belly. A few years ago he would have run out and had some more liposuction, but now he admits that what he really needs is a gym membership. He'll get one, he says, when he stops being lazy.

"Don't you think plastic surgery goes against naturalness?" asks Dorothy.

"Plastic surgery is about naturalness," says Fred. "Women don't want to have to wear heavy cosmetics." Fred has just a little foundation on. "They don't want their boyfriends to find out they have a different face when the makeup is removed. Women want to be like men in that sense. They want to go out bare-faced and scrubbed and look attractive. They don't want to paint it on. They don't want to take a shower at night and come out looking like the wrath of God. They want to know their look is always there.

"So many women are willing to look not as beautiful as they could for part of the day so they don't have to be let down when they wash their face. Years ago, women who weren't beautiful became very striking because of makeup. But when their faces came off at night, the person they were with...well, if it was true love it was one story, but if it was a first date, it would be something else."

Phyllis walks into the restaurant; she's joining a party of two. Her wig is off and she's wearing sunglasses.

Not many women can look regal while wearing sunglasses at night in a hotel in Oak Lawn, Illinois, but Phyllis does it. "She looks like somebody," says Dorothy.

"Beauty is more than surgery," Fred says. But Phyllis got great results because she started early. That's what Dolly Parton did, too. She said so in *TV Guide*: "I'd rather [have a lift] done every two years than wait too long, when all of a sudden everybody knows you've had a face lift. And you look so tight, like a banjo head."

"Beauty is also the way you move, the way you think, and finally the way you package yourself," says Fred. "You can look like a sixty-year-old woman, or you can look like a sixty-year-old woman who's had plastic surgery, or you can look like a woman who is sixty and looks as young as her plastic surgeon made her."

"What's the difference between the last two?"

"Phyllis and a woman who may have had good work but has no style and doesn't take care of herself," says Fred. "Phyllis works hard, honey. She does the treadmill every day, eats well, and drinks tons of water. And I get top-of-the-line, state-of-the-art beauty aids for her. I know a lot of women Phyllis's age who look like they could be her mother."

"But isn't surgery substituting for a more profound issue?" says Dorothy.

"If it is, how will you know until you have the work out of the way?" I say. "Plastic surgery's power is so overrated. Most surgery happens when a rich lady gets the snapshots back from her Greek vacation, sees she has a double-chin, and has the time and money to do something about it."

"Plastic surgery can ease you through a period of your life when you're getting depressed about aging," says Fred. "It won't get rid of the depression, but it can help ease you through. And if you choose to have surgery," he says, "you should like your surgeon and do what Phyllis does: Charm the guy, make him interested in how you look."

"Fred," I say, "it's easy for a celebrity billionaire to do that, but what about the rest of us? You're totally self-conscious when you go, and aren't in the mood to charm. And a lot of these guys don't seem to be very warm."

"That's true," says Fred. "They have huge egos and you are to shut up and let them do whatever they are to do to you, which is fine as long as they're going to be honest. This friend of mine in New York was fifty-two and looking great, but one day it started to happen," says Fred. "She was starting to look ten years older. She went to one of the best and he quoted her twelve thousand dollars.

"I told her, 'For that price, he's not going to do it. His assistant is going to do it once you are asleep. Tell him you want him to do it without anybody working on the side and you're willing to pay whatever the fee is.'"

"So what did he charge her?" Dorothy says.

"Twenty-three thousand dollars," says Fred. "And I told her to get it videotaped. And you know what? In five days that woman was in my chair getting makeup; that's how good a job he did. In three weeks her stitches were out and she had no scars.

"The racket," says Fred, "is when people get butchered. The surgeon starts, but when you're asleep the assistant takes over."

"But if almost everybody in Hollywood over age forty has had work done, why don't we see more botched jobs?"

"Makeup and lighting can save almost anything."

"What about those ladies with tight skin who blink too much?"

"It's dry-eye syndrome," says Fred. "The tear ducts have been damaged when the eyes have been pulled so far back. I've known women who had to tape their lids closed so they could sleep at night…. But the surgery is always getting better. Gloria Swanson and women from that era wore bangs to hide the scars from primitive plastic surgery. They used to pull from the forehead; now they pull from the side."

Still, Fred's all for it "when the inside of the individual needs to be portrayed more on the outside."

Fred looks at Dorothy. "If you play with your nose any more than clipping it here"—he touches her nose—"or giving it a little touch, you'll end up a Plain Jane. Your eyes are big. A little bit of makeup would make you look like a great beauty of your time."

"What time is that?" Dorothy asks.

"Your time," says Fred.

Fred suggests we go up to his room and work on Dorothy's face. Dorothy's smiling.

Fred puts on the fluorescent lights around his vanity mirror and looks at his reflection. "Ooooh," he says. "Harsh lights tell the truth, honey." He says he won't have any more work done, though. "My goal in my twenties was to have everything in place so when I aged, I would age gracefully. If I pulled my skin"—he pulls—"tight over my face, I'd look like a severe old queen. Besides, I've dealt with my mortality."

Dorothy looks in the mirror. "Your cheekbones are fabulous," Fred says. "It wouldn't take a makeover to make you photogenic. Your chin and jawline are good. Your lips are a little thin."

"I used to go like this to make my lips fatter." Dorothy pouts. "I'll never be an ideal."

"Not an ideal, no," says Fred. "But those girls come and go. When I have a woman like you in my chair after doing one of those pretty girls, I say to myself, 'What is she going to look like in her fifties compared to what *you're* going to look like?'"

I don't say anything. Fred has a different fairy tale for each beauty trip. For the women who had beauty in their youth, he assures them it can always be preserved, that there will always be glances from strangers. For the plain, he promises them they can be transfigured into swans, even if it takes decades.

What concerns me now is that Dorothy and I could spend the rest of our lives on this trip, still tormented by the time when beauty is its purest and matters most—our teens and twenties. Still hoping that the beautiful competitors from our youth are ugly now. Still waiting to hear someone use the same words Fred is using, that one day we'll look better than they do.

But the clichés about beauty that were lies during our youth are now becoming true at age thirty. Dorothy and I tried to believe our parents when they told us in high school, "Nobody's looking at you. It's all in your head that they're pointing and laughing." But then, people were pointing, the ugly were humiliated, and the beauties were having their moments.

Now, as we age, most of us do become less noticed as we walk the streets. Youth and beauty aren't meeting our eyes, they are searching for reflections of themselves.

Vanity never ends, but I've found that one of the good things about getting older is—to paraphrase Fitzgerald—that we (ideally) gravitate toward intelligence and good manners. Making the distinction between looking your best and looking beautiful, and deferring to youth in matters of beauty is, I think, both smart and gracious.

A photographer I know, Arne Svenson, was taking photographs of a handsome father and his beautiful son. The father, too, had been beautiful in youth and in one frame bowed to the son's beauty by having only his hand photographed next to the boy.

I'm not saying that only the young should be photographed, or that we can't be sexy and provocative as we age, or that there aren't those who look smashing even in their sixties. But the immediate comfort of being told that beauty is not about youth, that it is always within the reach of our mirrors, could leave Dorothy and me stalled and self-absorbed, obsessed with a dream that's passed us by.

Fred is putting a little color in Dorothy's cheeks, then adding a little mascara to her eyes. Dorothy says daily mascara applications are a pain unless somebody does it for you. Fred says she could get her eyelashes dyed, it makes life easier.

"So, Fred," says Dorothy, "you're saying my moment of glory is when everyone else is getting plastic surgery?"

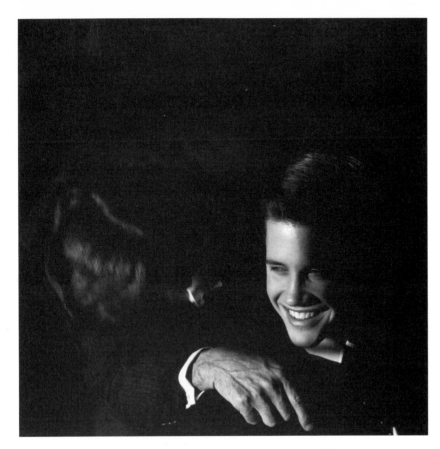

Father and Son
by Arne Svenson

"Your moment of glory could be tomorrow," says Fred. "When you put on a great Donna Karan suit, a little mascara, some clear lip gloss—you have thin lips, so why play with them—and strut down the street."

Fred takes out his hair spray, then rubs his fingers through Dorothy's hair. He wants every woman he touches to believe in magic.

When we get back to New York, Dorothy says, she's getting her lashes dyed. But we've got to see Ms. Olympia before we go home.

16

i have been on this trip for more than a year. I've never become bored looking at beauty, but it has been predictable to describe. The beauties have consistently been tall, thin young women with smooth skin who photograph beautifully. Or tall, thin women who photograph beautifully in part because their cosmetic surgery evokes youth. There are more ethnic beauties than before, but skin tone aside, they don't look much different from the Caucasians. The most radical look I've seen on the trip so far were Kristen NcMenamy's eyebrows.

There's nothing fair about beauty, but for men anyway, at least there's something of an equalizer: working out. When he was promoting *Rocky*, Sylvester Stallone said that as a kid he thought he didn't have any brains in his head, so he developed his body. For men, especially gay men, there's a similar philosophy: If you don't have a pretty face, you'd better get a buff body. It's a social survival instinct, a cold truism of gay life. Like women, gay men have to look good enough to catch the harshly critical eye of a male predator.

It took awhile for straight guys to get into the gym ritual. There were two things holding them back, white-collar guys especially. Muscles meant you were either working class (a Guido) or a vain primper (a homo).

But then weight training was taken up by more and more athletic programs as a strength builder, and Arnold Schwarzenegger became a superstar. Now straight guys could flex their muscles in front of each other in the locker room and discuss their diets without being called faggots.

"Fuck, man," I heard one guy say to another after a work out. "You're pumped. You wanna get something to eat?"

"All right, dude, but no pizza or beer. I'm workin' on my abs."

Americans have let themselves see that guys look better when they work out.

Now every soap opera has plots centered around the village hunk finding an excuse to take off his shirt.

"Your tropical fish need feeding, Anastasia? No prob, but I don't want to get fish water on this shirt, so…"

Weight training has become so mainstream in the last decade that shirtless men in magazines, TV, and movies are expected to have bodies sculpted by weights, to look no different from Greek kouroi.

But what happens when a woman wants to use the gym for weight training instead of aerobics class? And what if she isn't afraid to lift the maximum weight she can and in as many repetitions as possible?

The ancient Greeks and Romans recognized the beauty of female athletes and warriors— but with awe and fear. When the Greeks sculpted muscular Amazon warriors, they usually showed them wounded or dying because alive they were too much of a threat to men.

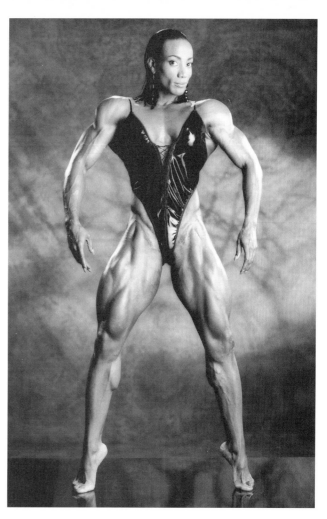

Lenda Murray
by Bill Dobbins

The bottom line is that female muscularity is genuinely threatening. To celebrate its beauty is genuinely radical. And when something radical starts to enter the mainstream, it upsets a lot of people.

Dorothy and I are on a flight to Los Angeles. She's looking through a copy of *Flex* magazine with Ms. Olympia, Lenda Murray, on the cover. All the photos of Lenda are by Bill Dobbins, the man we're flying to see. Bill cowrote *The Encyclopedia of Bodybuilding* with Arnold Schwarzenegger and is arguably the best bodybuilding photographer around. Lenda Murray is his muse.

"Oh my God," says Dorothy. "This is too much." Dorothy says she likes muscles on women, but muscles like Madonna has, or like Linda Hamilton had in *Terminator 2.* Ladylike definition. Only breasts should bulge in a woman, evidently. Not biceps.

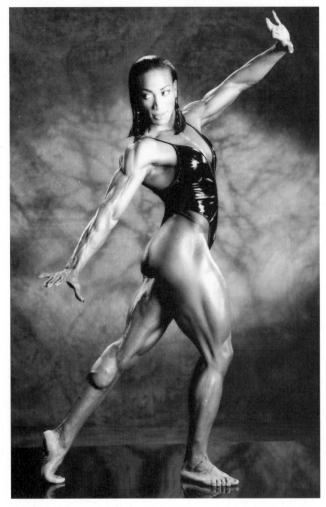

Lenda Murray
by Bill Dobbins

"Lenda's got a pretty face," says Dorothy, "but if you cover up the face and the breasts, that could be a man's body."

I hear it every time I show someone photos of Lenda. It's as if a preprogrammed tape goes off. I once wanted to write about female bodybuilders for a women's fashion magazine, but the editor said that was for trailer trash.

It's not that different from how people saw male bodybuilding a generation ago—at once intimidating and vulgar. The fashion world will probably never accept it, because female bodybuilders will never help them sell clothes—they look better with their clothes off than on. Female bodybuilders aren't for the Miss America Organization—they might frighten some of the other contestants and sponsors. A lot of *Playboy* models lift weights to stay toned, but female bodybuilders push straight guys' gender buttons as much as gay men do. If a woman can bench-press more than her boyfriend, what can she do to him in bed?

Like a lot of front yards in Los Angeles, Bill's has a sign that says he has an Armed Response alarm system installed in his home. Bill lifts weights; he's about six-foot-two, more than two hundred pounds. Dorothy and I thought he was forty from the looks of him. It turns out he's fifty.

Bill's got a couch and a chair in his living room. But other than that and some books, there's nothing here but his photos of male and female bodybuilders—framed and poster-sized. His photos reveal muscles that Dorothy and I never knew existed.

Bill started going to Gold's Gym in Venice when he was thirty years old. He was out of shape and skinny, only 140 pounds. It was the mid-seventies, just before *Pumping Iron* came out. Gold's Gym didn't have groupies or a clothing line yet; it was just a hole in the wall. But Schwarzenegger and all the greats trained there, and Bill—the only pencil neck around—trained beside them.

"I wasn't intimidated by Arnold and the rest because I wasn't competition and they weren't going to beat me up," says Bill. "I wasn't even on the same planet."

But Bill got on their good side. He'd been in radio, so he offered to do promos for the gym free of charge.

Then he hooked up with Arnold and they worked on some books together. Bill started taking bodybuilders' pictures, first of men, then of women.

"I am one of the few people in women's bodybuilding who didn't get involved because they were my type." But now they are extremely attractive to him. Bill wouldn't think of going out with a woman who lights up a cancer stick. And women like Jayne Mansfield, the type he was attracted to as a kid, seem out of shape to him today.

But most of America looks at what Bill photographs and says, "Freak show!"

Arnold Schwarzenegger
and Bill Dobbins
courtesy of Bill Dobbins

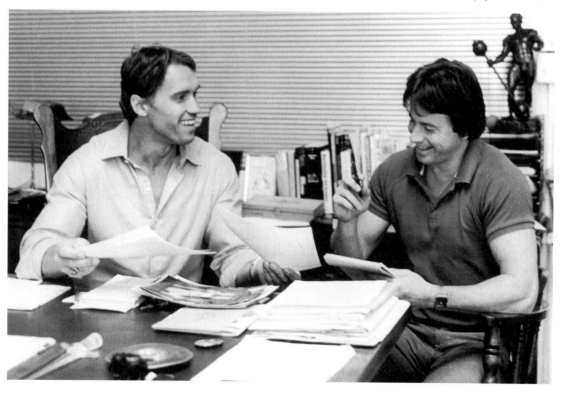

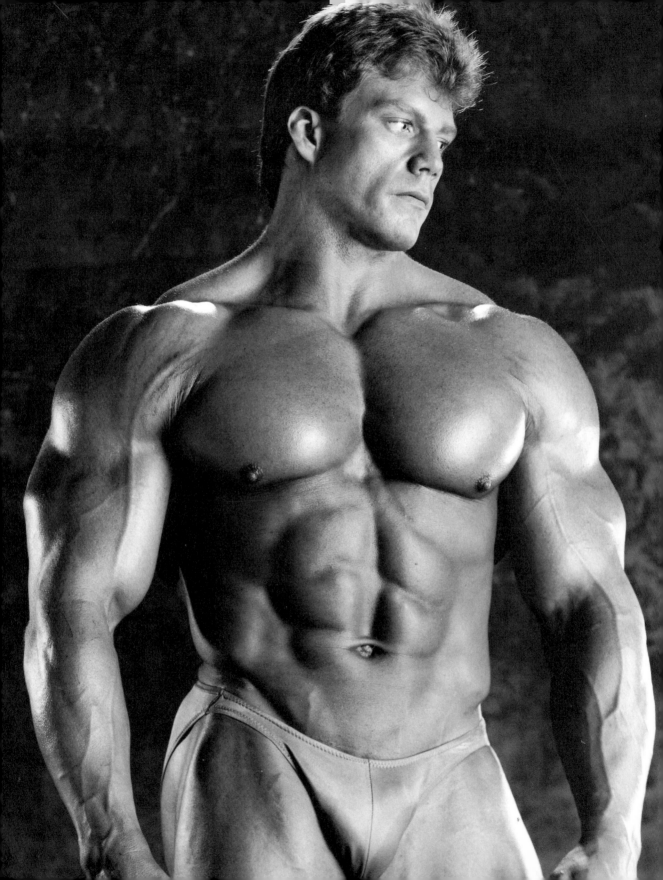

"There never have been women with muscles," says Bill. "Then again, there once never were women lawyers."

But like everybody says, It's *too much*. These women look like men.

"Stand a female bodybuilder next to Arnold and you'll see how small she really is," says Bill. "Her legs are the size of his arms."

"But that's not what scares people," I say. "What scares them is not when Lenda Murray stands next to Arnold, it's when Lenda stands next to the average American guy and could beat him up, no problem."

"Bodybuilding expands the spectrum of the way women can look," says Bill. "But you've got to realize that women aren't going to look like Lenda when they lift weights any more than men look like Arnold."

Lenda and Arnold couldn't have become champions if they hadn't been born with incredible genes. In that sense, they're no different from supermodels. The difference is that, unlike models, professional bodybuilders devote their lives to developing those genes. And the worldbeaters take steroids.

But bodybuilding is not about taking steroids and getting huge, Bill says. "Bodybuilding is a sport about the total aesthetic development of the physique. Just as opera isn't about singing loud, it's about singing beautifully." Critics who dwell on steroid use don't want to face the truth, says Bill, that the men and women he photographs have done something extraordinary with their bodies. Their destiny and discipline created something beautiful. Steroids only supplement that beauty. They do not create it.

In other words, steroids are to the best bodybuilders as morphine was to Poe, heroin was to Burroughs, acid was to the Beatles.... Would anyone who admires their work prefer they hadn't partaken? Should the people who use drugs to enhance their work have their work discredited because of it?

Is society willing to make a distinction between underage boys who take steroids so they can look pumped on the beach and adult bodybuilders who take them because they have a chance to make a living off their body?

That distinction has been made for Arnold. Even though he admitted taking steroids, he was still named America's fitness chief by President Bush and now has an advice column on health and fitness in *USA Today*.

But will a woman be forgiven?

Matt Mendenhall
by Bill Dobbins

Most men who lift weights at the gym a few times a week do not take steroids, obviously. But when they see a portrait of Arnold, they look at it with respect. They probably don't want to get that big (not that it's an option), but there's a macho instinct that also says there's nothing wrong with being that big. Guys pumped up with steroids at my gym are not pointed or laughed at, they are deferred to.

But when women see a portrait of Lenda, they often haven't decided if they should be trying to lift anything heavier than 10-pound dumbbells. So a woman who bench-presses 205 is beyond comprehension.

Bill finds my speculation tedious. "I'm dealing with the underlying truth, and when society comes around to understanding, that's fine," he says. "It would hardly be revolutionary if everybody agreed on this. If everybody understood this, we wouldn't be having this conversation."

Here's what's really interesting about bodybuilding, Bill says, and I don't interrupt: "We know the body deteriorates with age, but what would our quality of life be if we start bodybuilding at fifteen or eighteen? What is this going to do to our perception of the aging process when we have sixty-year-olds with the body of thirty-year-olds?

"To what degree should people be responsible for their own physical development? You don't feel sorry for the person whose teeth falls out because they don't brush or go to see a dentist. Does training become a responsibility?

"To what degree does the relative ease that women have been able to build muscle alter the way we look at the female physique? Of what femininity is? Then does this say all women should be muscular, or does this expand the way women can look?

"A lot of women have husbands who start looking around at other women at forty. If the wives had a body of a twenty-five-year-old, the husbands might still be hangin' in there."

Bill says that instead of women always saying they need to lose ten pounds and passively dieting, this is an aggressive and healthy way to go about looking their best. Bodybuilding (without steroids) can be just as transfiguring as cosmetic surgery, but without the risks.

"The average person doesn't listen to opera," says Bill. "They don't understand opera, but they respect it. What I want is for the average person to respect professional bodybuilding and some of them to like it.

"The big difference is you can admire Pavarotti, but he has nothing to teach you. But if you admire Lenda Murray, that may cause you to change the direction of your body. Bodybuilders have something to teach the public, not just inspire but actually teach them how to do something.

"Bodybuilding isn't the kind of beauty that fades—as long as you keep at it your whole life," says Bill. "It's one of the few areas where something done out of vanity produces results which are excellent to your health. But people will see what they want to see. They'll see what they expect to see. What they should be saying is, 'I'll see that when I believe it.'"

But what about those Calvin Klein ads? I ask. "Until I saw them, I didn't know a man's body could look that good."

"With female bodybuilding we're talking about something that will contradict your sense of reality," says Bill. "For you, the Calvin Klein ads were a heightened sense of reality. They were an ideal above what you expected, but not the opposite of what you expected. Female bodybuilding contradicts your sense of reality."

17

lenda Murray, Ms. Olympia, has to fix herself some breakfast, so Dorothy and I flip through her Victoria's Secret catalog while we wait.

On our flight here—L.A. to Detroit—Dorothy told me she'd wanted to feel the arms of Suzan Kaminga, a female bodybuilder she'd met at Bill's studio.

"I thought you said women bodybuilders are too masculine-looking," I'd said.

"I did." But once Suzan told Dorothy about the training she went through to get the body, Dorothy couldn't take her eyes off the physique.

"You mean you were more impressed by her training schedule than her body?"

"It was both," Dorothy said. "It was all so disciplined and healthy." What looked strange in photos felt strong and very sexual in the flesh. "People shouldn't trash female bodybuilders until they've sat next to one." Dorothy laughed.

Lenda has coffee black (with Equal) and oatmeal (390 calories, 7.4 grams of fat) with egg whites (51 calories, 0 fat) on top.

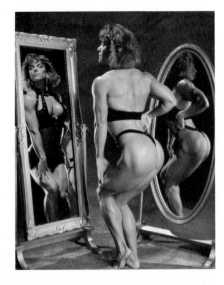

OPPOSITE:
*Lenda Murray
by Bill Dobbins*

BELOW: *Suzan Kaminga
by Bill Dobbins*

Lenda has to keep count of everything she consumes and all her measurements. She's two months away from the Ms. Olympia competition, where she's up for her fourth straight title.

Lenda is thirty-one, five-foot-five, and 149 pounds. Her body fat is 11 percent (7 percent at contest time) compared to 25 percent in most women. She doesn't starve herself; it's the opposite: she eats five meals a day. But none of the food is delicious. Lenda hasn't had a pizza in two years. It was a Hawaiian special, pineapple and ham.

Lenda has a ponytail and a high voice that says "That's so sweet" when she gets a compliment and "My goodness" when she's surprised. She looks more like a pretty jock with real big

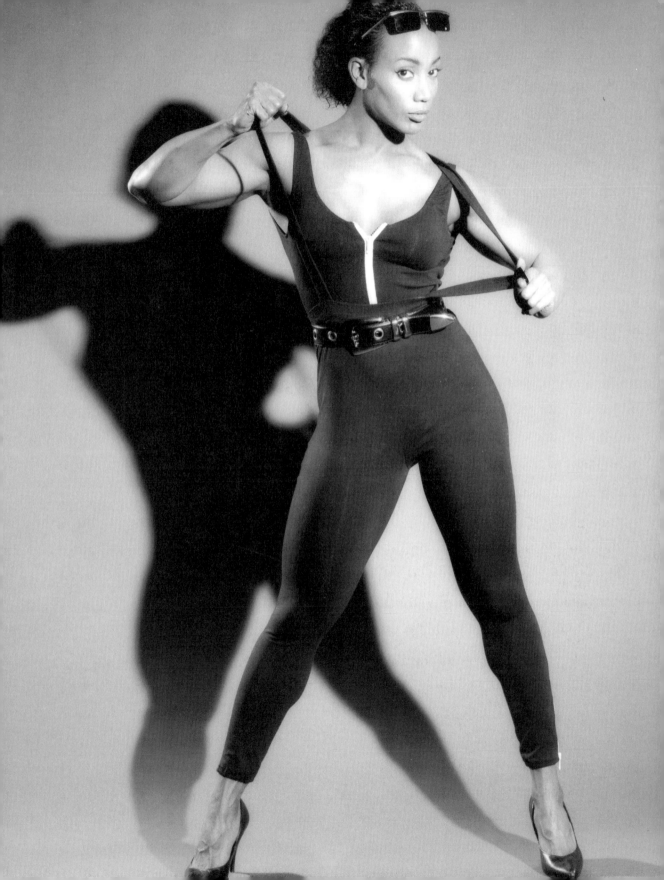

shoulders than the world's greatest female bodybuilder, but that's probably because her sweats are covering her arms.

Ten years ago, Lenda was one cut away from becoming a Dallas Cowboy cheerleader. It would have been the ultimate, she'd thought. "They were all so beautiful and glamorous." It was as far as a cheerleader could go, and Lenda has been cheering since high school. But she'd also run track and had beaten up the boys who tried to take lunch money away from her younger sisters. She was too muscular, the Cowboys said, so Lenda went home to Detroit to reduce for the final tryout.

Why was Lenda trying to get rid of what God had given her? That's what a Mr. Olympia competitor who trained at the same gym asked her. Didn't she realize that she had the potential to be a world beater?

Didn't he know? The Cowboy cheerleaders had a made-for-TV movie and their own lunch box.

Lenda lost some weight but not enough. So the day after she got back from Dallas, Lenda found that wise muscleman and never held back again, not with weights, anyway.

"Isn't that wild?" says Dorothy. "You went from the most stereotypically feminine role to the most revolutionary."

"That's right," says Lenda. "I'm glad the Cowboys cut me."

Lenda goes through her Victoria's Secret catalog with us. "I just can't wear something frilly or dainty," she says. "I've put on some dresses that make me look like a man in drag." She did find some clothes here, though, that she could order—stretchy and in medium. Sometimes Linda wishes she could have a bigger wardrobe, but she's usually in sweats, so it's just as well.

"These skinny models look great in clothes, but I don't think I would find them attractive in a swimsuit. When I look at their arms, I don't see the difference between the shoulder and the bicep and the tricep. Some of them look like they've dieted away their muscle."

Lenda finishes her oatmeal and egg whites.

"Do you ever miss Cream of Wheat with cheese?" I ask.

"I never had that. I miss fried shrimp the most." When Lenda gets cravings, she'll have a fat-free cookie or take a drive in her car on a sunny day.

Lenda's high-protein, low-fat meal plan is one of her daily beauty rituals. The others are aerobic and weight training, taking supplements, skin waxing, "creative music development" for her posing routine, the routine itself, and tanning. Even though she's black, tanning sessions are necessary to even her skin tone for competition. Lenda says she'll do as many of these rituals with us as possible today, although tanning is out of the question because only one individual is allowed per tanning bed.

Lenda also has to go to her accountant today for a Lenda Murray Inc. business meeting. She makes about $300,000 per year, most of it from endorsements.

While she trains for Ms. Olympia, Lenda moves out of her real house just outside of Detroit and lives in a condo with thick carpet, an unlisted number, and hardly any of her belongings. She doesn't want distractions. So we don't know what her taste in home furnishings is like, but Lenda says her favorite movie is *Amadeus* and she voted for Perot.

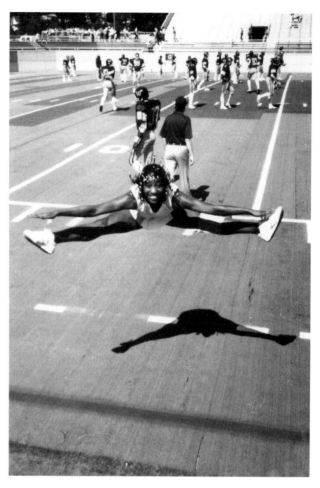

Lenda as cheerleader, courtesy of Lenda Murray

The condo has a mini-gym, and this is where Lenda does her first workout of the day—forty-five minutes of aerobics, half on the StairMaster and half on the bike. She says "Good morning" to everyone she sees; they're all in business suits and headed off to work.

Lenda works the StairMaster on full blast. Her foundation comes off on a white towel as she sweats, but she can carry on a conversation without running out of breath. The foundation wasn't concealing anything.

Lenda was raised in Detroit and she's been written up and been on the TV so much that most of the citizens are used to the sight of her now.

"Did Mayor Young proclaim a Lenda Murray Day?"

Parrillo Performance Diet Trac Sheet   Date _Oct 18_   Weight _149_

Time	Food and Quantity	Calories	Protein (grams)	Fat (grams)	Carbs (grams)	NA (mgs)	K (mgs)
8:00	Oatmeal (100)	**390**	14.2	7.4	64.2	2	352
	Egg Whites (100)	51	10.9	0	.8	146	139
	Cap-Tri (2)	228	0	0	0	0	0
		669	25.1	7.4	65.0	148	591
11:00	Cod (150)	117	26.4	.15	0	105	573
	Potatoe (200)	152	4.2	.2	34.2	6	814
	Brocolli (100)	32	3.6	.3	5.9	15	382
	Cap-Tri (2tb)	228	0	0	0	0	0
		529	34.2	.65	40.1	126	1769
1:00	Chicken (150)	175.5	35.1	2.85	0	75	480
	Brown Rice (50)	180	3.75	.95	38.7	4.5	107
	Corn (100)	96	3.5	1.0	22.1	0	280
	Green Beans	32	1.9	.2	7.1	7	273
	Cap-Tri (2)	228	0	0	0	0	0
		711.5	44.2	5.0	67.9	86.5	1110
3:00	Haddock (200)	158	36.6	.2	0	122	608
	Sweet Potato (200)	228	3.4	.8	52.6	20	486
	Brocoli (200)	64	7.2	.6	11.8	30	764
	Cap-Tri (2)	228	0	0	0	0	0
		678	47.2	1.6	64.4	172	1858
7:00	Pro-Carb (2 scoops)	210	8.0	0	44.0	128	344
8:00	Chicken (150)	175.	35.1	2.85	0	75	480
	Brown Rice (50)	180	3.75	.95	38.7	4.5	107
	Green Beans (200)	64	3.8	.4	14.2	14	486
	Cap-Tri (2)	228	0	0	0	0	0
		647.	42.6	4.2	52.9	93.5	1073
	TOTAL →	3444.	201.	18.8	334	754	6745

Lenda says she was about to get a key to the city, but Mayor Young's body-guard is her ex-boyfriend, and she's sure he told the mayor to give it to a visiting dignitary like Barbara Eden instead.

But the town BMW dealer gave her a BMW practically free of charge, so Lenda let him put a photo of her in his showroom.

Lenda always knew she was going to do something great, but she wasn't sure what it would be. She liked the pop icons of her time—Michael Jackson and Farrah Fawcett-Majors—but she didn't get her inspiration from them. She always went on instinct.

Lenda was one of the best athletes in her school, but since she was a girl the most recognition she could get was as a cheerleader, and even then she had to sell candy bars to pay for her uniform. Girls weren't allowed to use the weight room, but Lenda "once snuck into the forbidden room and felt instantly comfortable. I didn't need anybody to tell me how to work the machines."

Lenda studied political science at Western Michigan and kept cheerleading. Senior year, she cheered for the Michigan Panthers of the old USFL. When the Cowboys didn't hire her, she got a job in the human resources department of Burroughs Computers in Detroit. She always wore a suit so her muscles didn't show.

Lenda did not take steroids when she started training. "I'm glad I didn't," she says. "I never abused them, which is why I never got hair on my face or started talking like a man.

"But after the fourth year, when I won the state, I kept looking at other women and wondered how they got that lean and ripped and muscular. And it was explained to me that this [steroids] is what the top women do. I did want to get to the next level. So I actually did it. I've never abused it to the point that a lot of people think. When they look at us they think, 'All drugs.' Like right now? There's nothing in me. There can't be before a competition. And that's where genetics and hard work come to play. Because all those women who had been doing drugs from the start usually fall during this period. [Steroids alone] aren't going to make you a great bodybuilder, and to be honest I wish it had never been introduced to women."

So Lenda had a choice. She could have settled for being the best bodybuilder in Michigan and gone back to monitoring personnel files, or she could take

"What Lenda Ate Today,"
courtesy of Lenda
Murray

steroids and have a chance to become the best in the world at what she loved.

Lenda will never have to hide her body in a business suit again.

But that's not to say it never gets ugly, even since she became Ms. Olympia. She'll be in a line at the A&P with her brussels sprouts and cod "and the people behind me will start talking about steroids. I ignore them. It bothers them a lot more than if I talk back.

"What really bothers them is that I'm a woman who says something positive without opening my mouth. I'm strong and I've taken control of my life and I'm going to look the way I want to look, not the way they want me to look. They have to look in the mirror and see all the things they haven't done in their life. Maybe not bodybuilding, of course, but they know I've spent a lot of work and dedication to look this way."

Lenda's is such an American success story that I'm surprised I'm not in a line to interview her. Shouldn't she have been on the cover of *Ms.* by now and at least made an appearance on a Bob Hope Christmas special?

When Lenda is on TV, she gets asked a lot of downright rude questions. One waterhead asked her right off the bat, "Men don't find you attractive, do they?"

"How am I supposed to answer a question like that?" Lenda says to Dorothy and me. "Well, I get propositioned all the time."

I remember when Arnold was on a late-night Geraldo Rivera TV show in the seventies—years before Arnold became a movie star and married a Kennedy.

"Aren't all bodybuilders gay?" Geraldo asked.

Arnold just smiled, puckered up, and gave Geraldo a big old kiss.

But Lenda can't finesse the femininity issue with that kind of flippant charm. It's a lot more complicated. If Lenda is stronger than the average man, makes more money, and pursues a classic V-shaped male physique, what's left to be feminine?

Breasts, a pretty face, and being able to have a baby are the first things that come to my mind.

Lenda has silicone breast implants. She doesn't worry about them, because if something happens, there's always something else worse, she says. Ever since she was a teenager, she "always wanted to have breasts. Athletic women are so low in body fat we hardly have any."

Lenda had some minor work done to her face. She got rid of a bump on her nose. "I want a black person's nose," she says, "but without a bump." She also got rid of her overbite.

"To be honest," she says, "there are certain things that maybe I wouldn't have done, but when you look at yourself in the magazines and are photographed from every angle over and over and you see every flaw and people comment on those flaws…"

"I know how painful a snapshot can be," I say. "So being photographed at every angle all the time must be like living in a three-way mirror with fluorescent lighting."

"That's right," she says.

Does Lenda want to have a baby?

"I was thinking about that last night. I was just trying to imagine myself pregnant. It would be tough to compete if I had kids. But maybe I could be like Florence Griffith-Joyner, be the first to win an Olympia after having a baby."

But before she has a baby, Lenda has to work things out with her man. Derrick is an engineer. He used to be her fiancé, but now he's just her boyfriend.

Lenda drives Dorothy and me to her weight-training gym, Powerhouse. When in doubt, she always gives the other driver the right of way.

Lenda will work with weights here for around an hour and fifteen minutes. And she'll do forty-five more minutes of aerobic activity at her condo gym before she goes to bed tonight.

Powerhouse is almost empty now, but the funny thing is, says Lenda, when it gets crowded, guys think they should give her advice, even though she's won bodybuilding's greatest title three years in a row.

"Could you imagine them doing that to Lee Haney [Mr. Olympia]?" says Lenda. "Guys come up to me and want to show me how to train, tell me what to eat. They even approach me when I'm in the middle of a set."

"That's the male fuckin' ego," says Dorothy.

Lenda's always polite to interrupting men, but makes clear that it's dangerous to interrupt someone when she's about to hoist 200 pounds.

Lenda can bench-press 205, but she usually does 180 in reps of eight. She can squat up to 315; today she does 250, also in reps of eight.

It's strength, fitness, and beauty for the sake of strength, fitness, and beauty. Lenda is less a role model than an inspiration.

Dorothy watches how smoothly Lenda works out and swears she'll join a gym when we get back to New York.

The space where Lenda does her posing is booked, so we're going to watch *Oprah*. Diana Ross is plugging her autobiography, *Secrets of a Sparrow*.

Lenda says she can relate to a lot of what Diana is talking about. It's hard for a man to deal with a strong woman.

"What kind of man do you want, Lenda?"

"I like athletic men."

"But do you want to be stronger than him physically?"

"I would want him to be stronger than me because men are naturally stronger."

"Well, what if he's athletic but still isn't as strong as you?"

"That wouldn't be a problem for me. If there's a problem, it would be with him."

A guy was once hitting on Lenda in an airport. He said, "I don't know about you, your arms are bigger than mine," and Lenda said, "Well, whose fault is that?"

"If things don't work out with Derrick, would you want to date professional bodybuilders?"

A bodybuilder's physique appeals to her, but in her ten years of bodybuilding she's not met one who's been date bait.

"It's impossible to deal with their egos," Lenda says. "They're God, and women are nothing. The bodybuilders' wives are like 'Oooh, I cook all his meals and follow him all around.' Don't they want a woman with brains, one who is challenging?"

"Lenda, do you want a man to play that servant role for you?"

"Not at all."

Lenda thinks Derrick keeps tabs on her, and it's irritating. She checks the parking lot to see if he's outside.

"It's like Diana Ross said," says Lenda. "Men always want more control. Derrick doesn't have a problem with my muscularity, but he does have problems with the sport and the attention it brings me."

"I guess it is hard," I say. "I mean, your being an object of desire and all."

Lenda says she is her own business, Lenda Murray Inc., so people call her all the time wanting to buy her posters and T-shirts. When a man calls, a fan or a journalist, Derrick often says, "Who was that on the phone?" and Lenda will say, "I don't know," and he'll say, "What do you mean you don't know, he's callin' you at home."

Derrick does not like the idea of other men doing those sexy portraits of Lenda, so she hides a gothic drawing Boris Valejo did of her for his 1995 calendar underneath the sofa cushion. She knows that picture will upset Derrick.

"Would you pose in *Playboy*?" Dorothy asks.

"I'm very comfortable with my body, but I'd never want to have pictures taken with my legs spread open. I don't think it would be demeaning if it was a picture that showed off my muscular physique."

"Yours could be the first *Playboy* photo that men could fantasize about and women could put on their refrigerator for inspiration," says Dorothy.

"That's right," says Lenda.

The phone rings. Lenda says it's probably Derrick checking up on her, but it turns out to be her father. He just got discount air tickets to New York for the Ms. Olympia contest. The whole family's going, her parents and her sisters, Stacy, Cynita, Brenda, and LaTito.

"Is that after Tito Jackson?" I ask.

"I don't know. My father threw that 'La' in there."

"I hope it never comes to this," I say, "but what if you had to choose between a man and this career?"

"I think about my parents and my sisters and how hard my father had to work [compared to] the amount of money I've made in a short period of time," Lenda says. "I got a lot of strength and motivation from my parents. I realize people look up to me. I realize that there are a lot of black women who probably know nothing about bodybuilding but they can be sitting down and I'm on TV and seeing me lets them know that they can go out and get that college degree or lose that twenty to fifty pounds. I definitely would sacrifice a love life right now for that because my responsibilities are bigger than when I first started. I want to be in love, to be with someone, but I'm the one in the family now who has the opportunity, and I have to do as much as I can with it. I hope it doesn't turn out that way, but I am willing to sacrifice a love life for this."

We go to the mall to get Lenda a copy of Diana Ross's autobiography. Lenda's wearing jeans and a red pullover that has long sleeves but hugs her body. So she even gets more attention than the mall employees who are handing out free samples of food.

Lenda admits she'll miss all the attention when she retires, but she'll probably try to go for a few more Ms. Olympia titles first.

Bill Dobbins wants Lenda to move to Los Angeles. He says it will be good for her career. Maybe she can become an actress. Still, Lenda's going to stay in Detroit for now.

"I want to work with kids. I'll teach them what I've learned, that there's something better out there."

We're standing in a checkout line at the bookstore. A chubby teenaged clerk who's been watching Lenda comes to her and says, "How did you get shoulders like that? How do you do that?"

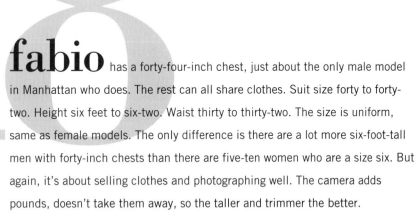

18

fabio has a forty-four-inch chest, just about the only male model in Manhattan who does. The rest can all share clothes. Suit size forty to forty-two. Height six feet to six-two. Waist thirty to thirty-two. The size is uniform, same as female models. The only difference is there are a lot more six-foot-tall men with forty-inch chests than there are five-ten women who are a size six. But again, it's about selling clothes and photographing well. The camera adds pounds, doesn't take them away, so the taller and trimmer the better.

There are some distinguished older gentlemen models, but youth is beauty. Almost any male model can easily be styled to look like a beautiful fraternity boy.

A male model lives one flight above me, in the penthouse apartment. His ads are always in the newspapers and magazines. I want to talk to him about beauty, but he has a girlfriend and I'm afraid if I brought up the subject in the elevator or laundry room, he'll think I'm making a pass. So I look him up in the Wilhelmina Men catalog (Josh, 6'1", 40L), and write to him, care of his agent.

"I'd like to help you out, man," he says, "but I don't have anything to say about beauty. If it was real estate or music you wanted to talk about..."

I call Dorothy. She told me once that a lot of male models who pose in *Playboy* fashion spreads come to her office. Does she know any?

Not really.

"How about the guys you work with, do they ever talk about male beauty?"

BELOW: Josh
by Mikael Jansson

OVERLEAF: Sy Sperling
by Steve Napolitano
and Michel Delsol

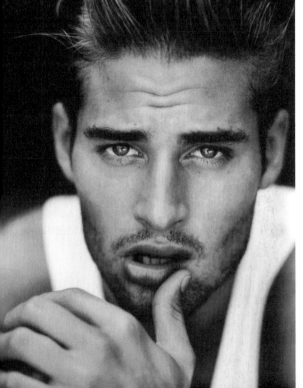

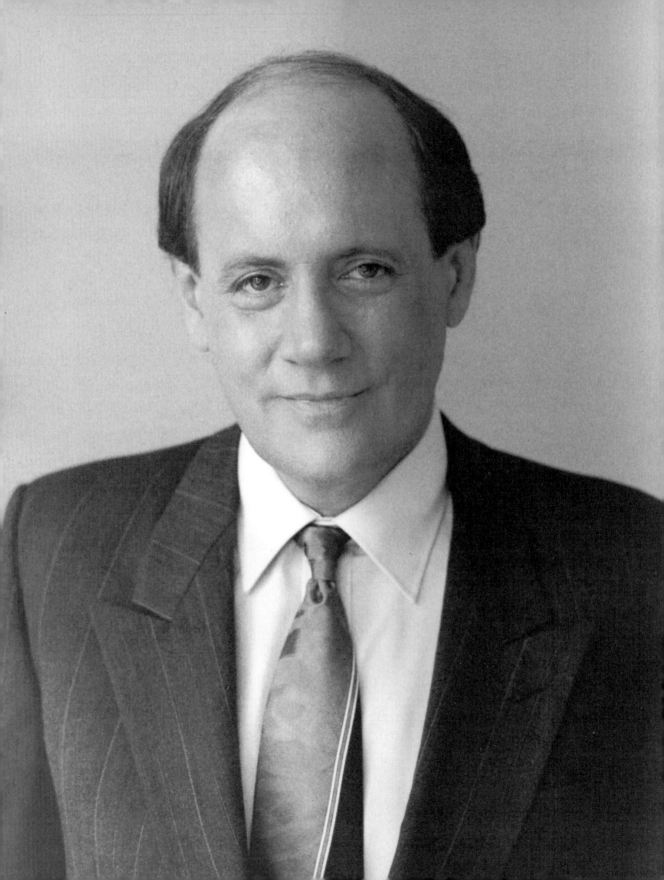

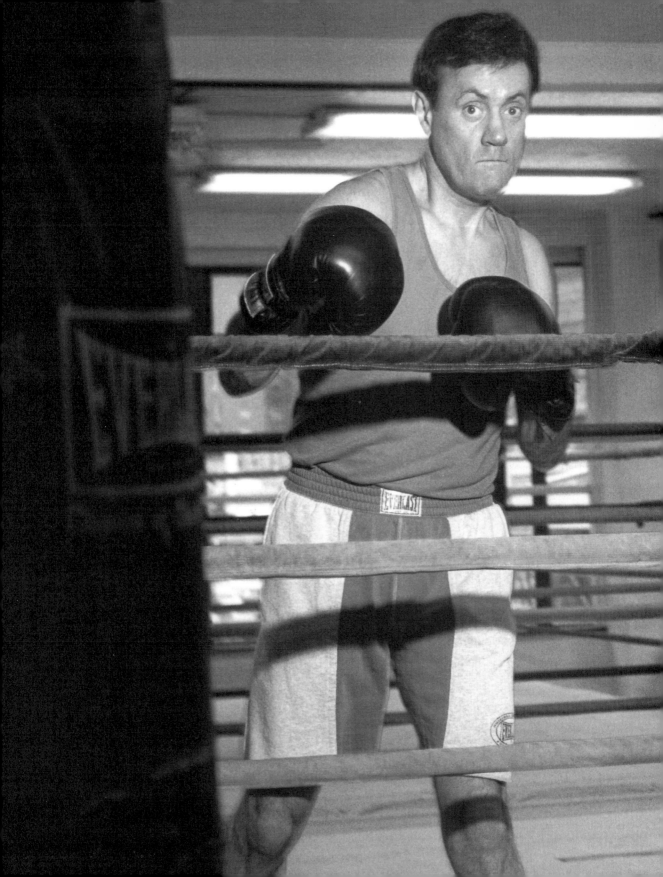

"All the guys here are straight, and all they'll admit to wanting is a flat stomach and a full head of hair."

So I figure Sy Sperling is a straight man who would be comfortable talking—if
not about male beauty, at least about all the beautiful male hair he has for sale.

Sy is the businessman who was unself-conscious enough to make a TV commercial that showed viewers he's a chrome dome who happens to wear a rug, I
mean, a hair-replacement system. "I'm not only president of the Hair Club for
Men," he said. "I'm also a client." It was the most successful before/after ad
since that skinny guy bought a Charles Atlas muscle kit and stopped getting
sand kicked in his face.

Sy tells Dorothy and me he never worried about getting beaten up on account
of being so tough that he was in a Bronx gang called the Golden Guineas, even
though he was Jewish. "I was considered the toughest guy in the school, the
toughest guy in the neighborhood, probably the toughest guy in the region—the
entire North Bronx region."

This was the 1950s, before gangs started using guns, but Sy would pull out a
knife if he had to. But now that Sy has so much money that he's appeared on
Lifestyles of the Rich and Famous, he'd back away from a fight. If Sy whupped
someone who got a look at his famous head, he'd be sued big time.

Sy's a strict vegetarian now, and there's no meat or dairy allowed at this
restaurant. If you want cream in your coffee, it's BYO. Dorothy and I order the
vegetarian duck and share.

Sy is wearing his hair-replacement system. Dorothy says it looks real to her
and that Sy is taller, more confident and handsome than he appears on TV.

I look at Sy's system and wonder about my own hair. I've always hoped that
since I was so plagued by acne, fate would kindly spare me baldness. But I
worry because my father has lost most of his hair. Then again, my uncle—my
mother's brother—collects social security and still has a full head of hair. It's as
black as Ronald Reagan's was when he was in office.

If I do go bald, I'm sure I'd consider purchasing Sy's product. It does fit well
on Sy, but I'm afraid I would always be self-conscious if I was wearing it, probably feeling the same way I did when I wore foundation (Clinique, porcelain
beige). Whenever people looked at me, I wasn't sure if they were admiring my

outfit or thinking that my makeup wasn't blended properly. Likewise, if I had on someone else's hair, I'd be afraid that it would either fall off or I'd run into the person who used to own it.

"Sy, where does the hair you use come from?"

"India," he says.

"Dead people?"

"Ken, gross," says Dorothy.

"No," says Sy. It's from people who evidently have long hair and a notion to sell it, like the lady in the O. Henry story, "Gift of the Magi." Sy says the hair is anonymous, so clients can't communicate or become pen pals with the people whose hair they are wearing.

Does Sy go to India and check all the hair out himself? No, but if you look in the Yellow Pages under hair supplies, you'll find wholesalers who sell human hair by the pound. Since Sy practically buys by the ton and has a lot of leverage in the business, he gets the choicest stuff.

But everybody in India has black hair, and guys in Sy's commercials are blond, brunette, even some carrot tops.

"The hair is dyed," says Sy.

Sy's father was a bald-headed Bronx plumber. He had "the Bozo look," says Sy. "He allowed the side of his hair to grow and that accentuated the baldness." He was bothered by it enough to rub his scalp with wintergreen oil. It smelled up the house worse than limburger cheese, but Sy's dad swore it was making his hair sprout. Sy was a good son and would say, "Yeah, Dad, right, it's true. That's a true statement."

The baldness didn't bother Sy's mother, though. She was more concerned about his making a living. "She was very practical, like most Jewish mothers."

Sy was very looks conscious as a teenager. Like his dad, he had a hair-loss problem early in life. He had a high forehead, plus thinning hair to boot (you could see his scalp when he used Brylcreem). That's why the young people called him Chrome Dome.

"Sometimes I'd look in the mirror and say to myself, 'You know, I have pretty good features,' but for some reason when I flirted with women, I was very unsuccessful and I never really knew why."

Sy would get turned down at social events when he asked women to dance. The neighborhood girls wouldn't go out with him. "They loved me like a *broth-uh*," says Sy. "Everybody loved me like a *brothuh.*"

Sy knew it wasn't all about looks. It was class, too. He had moved from "the Bronx ghettos" to a more middle-class neighborhood. The girl he fancied, Sharon Finkelstein, wanted to go out with guys who were going to be doctors or lawyers. Sy didn't know about the hair-fusion method then, he didn't have a five-year career plan, so he went to the air force after high school.

He boxed a lot and beat up several pilots in the ring. Sy says he defeated the eighth-ranked heavyweight of the world in a three-round match. "I couldn't have beaten Ali," he says. "But I probably could have beaten Patterson, Quarry...." Still, Sy saw what happened to a lot of boxers and didn't want to become an idiot with a caved-in head. Boxing was out as a career option. He started selling pools and carpets and purchased a rug to make himself more appealing. The product turned into a hair ball when Sy wore it in the shower, and it took almost two hours to untangle.

In 1968, Sy created one of his first hair-replacement systems and put it on his father's head. It didn't fit, and the old man accused his son of giving him a secondhand hairpiece. Not much later, his father passed away.

"When women say hair loss doesn't bother them, what they mean is they're not going to divorce a guy they're married to if he's losing his hair," says Sy. "But when a guy with a full head of hair approaches a woman in a bar, she's more likely to talk to him than to a guy who's balding."

It's really simple when you think about it, says Sy, like a formula: "If a guy is twenty-five and doesn't have hair on top, why would a twenty-three-year-old woman talk to him if he looks forty, when she can talk to someone who looks her own age?"

Sy is fifty-two. Not too long ago, he separated from his wife, Amy, who invented the Hair Club strand-by-strand system that Sy's now wearing. They're still friends, but Sy hit the singles bars until he met his new girlfriend:

"Now, if I didn't have hair, I'd probably be talking to women forty to fifty. But I [wore hair] and I met my girlfriend, who's thirty-six years old and very attractive, very charming, and we have a great relationship. I'm sure if I didn't look youthful to her she wouldn't have talked to me the first night we met."

"But, Sy," Dorothy says, "you're a celebrity. Of course women want to meet you."

"I don't want women to be attracted to me because I'm a wealthy entrepreneur," says Sy. "I'm not a bald, fat celebrity. I'm somebody who is well groomed. If Don Rickles went to a club, they might want his autograph, but I don't know how well he'd do socially. Besides, I didn't become famous because I broke the four-minute mile or I won the Nobel prize. I'm famous because I made a commercial. I paid for my own celebrity. So what's the big deal?"

"It's still celebrity," I say. "What gives you more confidence—fame or hair?"

"I want to have sex appeal, I want to be able to relate to a woman thirty-five years old. I want to market myself so that I can appeal to a woman who is two decades younger. I want to have as much appeal as possible in the same way [I want my ads] to appeal to as many people as possible."

Whenever they get the chance, men go for youth and beauty.

"At least he's being honest about it," Dorothy whispers to me.

But when does it end? If you're an older man—but rich or famous—you will probably always be able to attract youth and beauty until you keel over.

"Do you think that maybe you'd have stayed with your wife if you'd stayed bald?" I want to say: "Did your new hair and fame distract you from the real thing?" but I don't because how do I know how real his marriage was?

Sy says if he'd never gotten hair, then he'd be more unhappy with himself and "very insecure with my wife. I would have made her miserable. I would have been getting on her case, you know. 'Why are you looking at that guy?'"

"What do you think of hair in a can?" I ask. "You know, the stuff you spray on your bald spot?"

Sy says it's nothing compared to what Hair Club can do.

"My commercial changed the way people think. At one time wearing any kind of artificial hair was considered to be an embarrassment. I removed the shroud of secrecy. Here I am bald, here I am with hair, there's nothing wrong with it." Sy didn't remove his hair during dinner to make the point.

"We were the first to offer a nonsurgical semipermanent type of hair replacement. You never hear the word toupee anymore, it's an anachronism."

Sy hates bad hair jobs. They stand out like a sore thumb and give his busi-

*Rudy Giuliani
by Stephen
Kroninger/Village Voice*

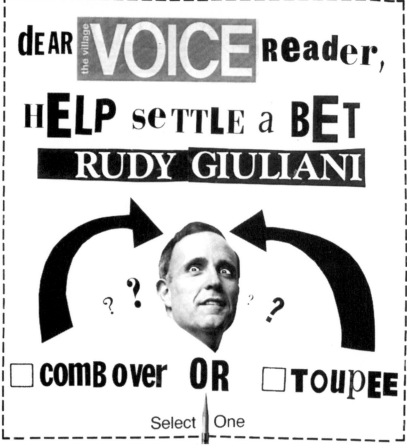

ness a bad name. "I'd pay Howard Cosell not to wear a piece," says Sy.

A lot of style-conscious Manhattan liberals had a problem voting for Mayor Giuliani because he was a Republican and they didn't like his haircut. What was the deal? Was it a toupee or a comb-over?

Sy says he gave money to Giuliani's campaign the first time he ran for mayor, but not the second.

"If I write his campaign a check again, I want to get something in return, and that would be fun for him to become a client and give us a testimonial. So if somebody says to him, 'Hey, Rudy, your hair looks terrific,' he would say, 'Hair Club is my stylist.' I don't want to promote a guy who is promoting the bald or covered look. I'm very pragmatic as a businessman. I don't want people thinking this guy is a client. One hand washes the other. I want him to be a client of ours because he looks like he's a bad client of ours now."

I ask Sy about beautiful guys, the ones in Bruce Weber photos and Calvin Klein ads with perfect faces and pecs.

"Over ninety percent of the male public does not have an interest in that," says Sy.

Sy will admit to hair envy, going to the gym to keep his body fit, even to getting the bags under his eyes removed. He wants to look good, but isn't tortured by not being an ideal. And he's not interested in discussing the ideal, either. That's for the other ten percent of the "male public"—mostly gay homosexuals like me—to agonize over.

"A lot of people who know me think of me as an anomaly," says Sy. "What do you think of me? Sometimes you question where you fit in the universe."

"You're very on the table," says Dorothy, and I nod.

19

when i was a pizza-faced teenager in the seventies, I was so hard up for a glimpse of male beauty that I'd stare at the Dads and Lads underpants section of the Sears catalog. I'd shoplift copies of *Seventeen* because only girls were supposed to think Shaun Cassidy was cute. I'd position myself in the cafeteria so I could see the biceps of the school hunk expand when he brought a meaty sandwich to his lips.

Marky Mark in Times Square by Michel Delsol

Now I wonder why I almost flunked Greek history in high school, the same class where slides of sculpted Greek men were flashed to us on audio-visual day. How come our teacher didn't talk about the cult of the beautiful boy in Greek art? It's probably because he could have gotten himself fired, as we lived in the state that elected Jesse Helms.

But it wasn't just the Bible Belt. It turns out that in the early to mid-seventies, Bruce Weber was taking photos of the same type of beautiful guys he shoots today and was told he'd never be a success, that nobody outside SoHo and Greenwich Village would want to see his work.

But in the late seventies, Arnold Schwarzenegger and Lou Ferrigno made it okay for straight guys to show off their muscles. High school and college boys would put Ferrigno's *Incredible Hulk* posters on their walls. And when *American Gigolo* came out in 1980, Richard Gere had muscles that weren't cartoonish. The male body could be sculpted with aerobics and weights instead of steroids and weights. And he had a pretty face.

In 1982, Calvin Klein and Bruce Weber made the pretty hunk a commercial deity. Weber's photo of a tanned, muscular pretty boy in Calvin Klein underpants was little different from the work he'd been doing for years. But now it was on a gargantuan billboard in Times Square and in full-page magazine ads.

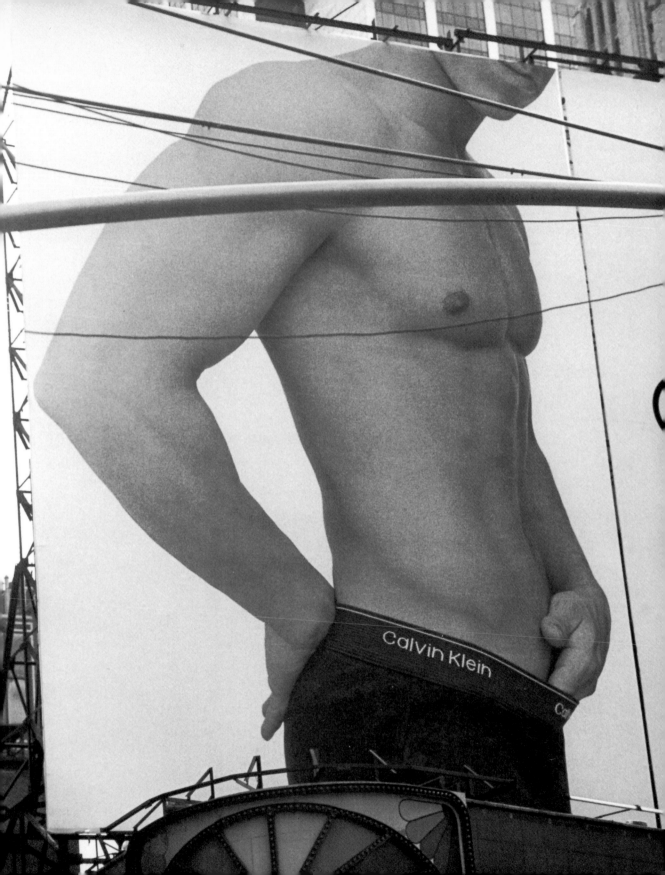

Now I—and other gay men—didn't have to purchase teen-dream or physique rags to ogle our ideal, women could see how their men came up short, and straight guys—if only for a second—were forced to contemplate bisexuality.

Weber's and Klein's beauty was new in American pop culture, but not art history or gay culture. It did not create a new kind of beauty but did heighten awareness of it. In other words, if Montgomery Clift were around today, he'd be provided with a personal trainer to enhance his shirtless scenes.

Weber's work is American pop culture at its best because it did what Greek sculpture and museums failed to do: It got middle America to appreciate the beauty of the male physique. But even the most seductive ad campaign can't change the lasting imbalance of the beauty trip. A guy who sees a Calvin Klein model in Times Square might feel a tug of inadequacy, but he's not going to torture himself for not being that ideal, unless women start looking at men the same way Sy Sperling looks at women. Will wives ever start saying to their husbands, "Keep eating beer with doughnuts, lard-ass, and I'm outta here? There's a tasty dish at the gym whose squats make me quiver"?

Dorothy says, "That won't work because hot young guys don't want divorcées. They want young girls or other hot boys." There are always exceptions, she says. "But it's an animal instinct and it's not going to change."

Around the same time the first Calvin Klein hunk was unfurled in Times Square, I started studying Andy Warhol's *Interview* magazine, especially the photos by Bruce Weber and Christopher Makos. By the time I moved to New York City in 1986, I had learned the beauty rules of Warhol, pop culture's most famous aesthete:

1. If you don't have a beautiful face, get a buff body, preferably with the help of a beautiful personal trainer. (I joined a gym, but couldn't afford a personal trainer.)

2. Correct facial flaws with as many beauty products and collagen injections as possible. (I do not look good in foundation, but I did visit all the plastic surgeons.)

3. Try to become famous because fame attracts beauty. It is the one thing that can catch the eye as instinctively and quickly as beauty does. (I can't

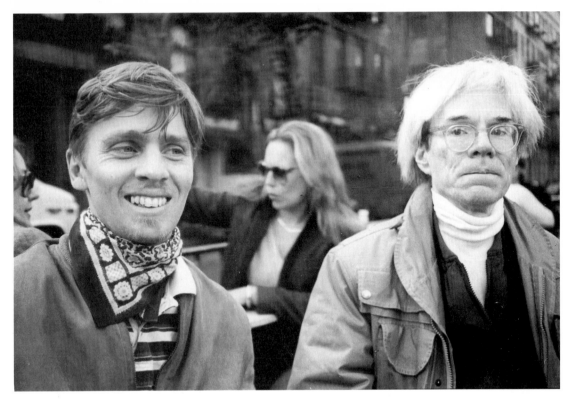

*Christopher Makos and
Andy Warhol
by Christopher Makos*

sing or dance and I snuck out of acting lessons when the teacher asked the
class to form a circle, join hands, and counter-clockwise, say something good
about the thespian standing next to us. All I could do was write a novel. It
didn't bomb, but it didn't make me famous, either. Besides, by the time it
was published, Andy Warhol had died.)

But his protégé, Christopher Makos, is still around.

Christopher drove to New York City in a Mustang, all the way from
California. Christopher's not good with exact dates, but it was the early seventies and he was in his early twenties, a blank slate, he said. One of his former
boyfriends, the writer Dotson Rader, told me Christopher was "one of the great
American beauty roses of his generation. I still have a photo of him as a
teenager and it's enough to make you weep."

Christopher hooked up with Tennessee Williams in no time and became his
assistant. And not much later, Christopher was traveling the world with Andy
Warhol, taking photos of Warhol with all the beautiful people.

Christopher survived being a beautiful boy for famous people. He's forty-

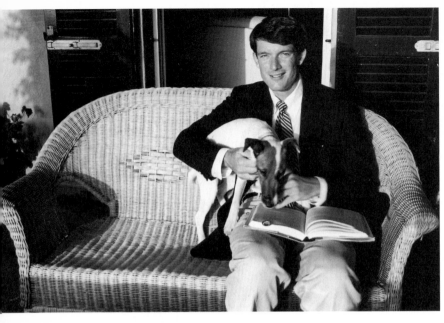

six now and has his own photo studio with his portraits of Warhol, Elizabeth Taylor, and his "Davids": all-American white bread, aged eighteen to twenty-five, with muscles and no shirts.

Christopher goes to the gym. He has a lot of hair, a flat stomach, and a personal trainer whom he also photographs. But Christopher's not happy when he has to pose for photos now; he gets real impatient. He trav-

ABOVE: *Paul Washington by Christopher Makos*

OPPOSITE: *Paul Washington's legs by Christopher Makos*

OVERLEAF, LEFT: *Morgan Winsor by Christopher Makos*

OVERLEAF, RIGHT, CLOCKWISE FROM TOP LEFT: *Brian Smith, Michael Loomis, Andrew Vitrano and Pat Scarlet by Christopher Makos*

els in the same circles he always did, but not as the object.

His "close friend and muse," Paul Washington, is so good-looking that Christopher has known him for over a year and hasn't lost the desire to photograph him just about every week. The guy's a real golden boy. He's going to law school now, and he has the kind of charm that makes me think if he's running for something, I'll vote for him.

I ask Christopher if he'd ever had a relationship with someone who was neither beautiful nor famous.

No, not really.

"What's the difference," I ask him, "between how you look at beautiful guys compared to the way Tennessee and Warhol did?"

Christopher thinks Tennessee was tortured by beauty, not because he wasn't a beauty rose himself, but because of the times. In Tennessee's day, you could get electroshock therapy if you were a guy who talked too much about how good-looking Montgomery Clift was.

Warhol had hang-ups similar to Tennessee's, Christopher says, but by the time Christopher and Warhol were traveling together in the late seventies, male beauty could be discussed openly. Not only that, Christopher taught Warhol that beautiful boys—especially actors and models—were more than

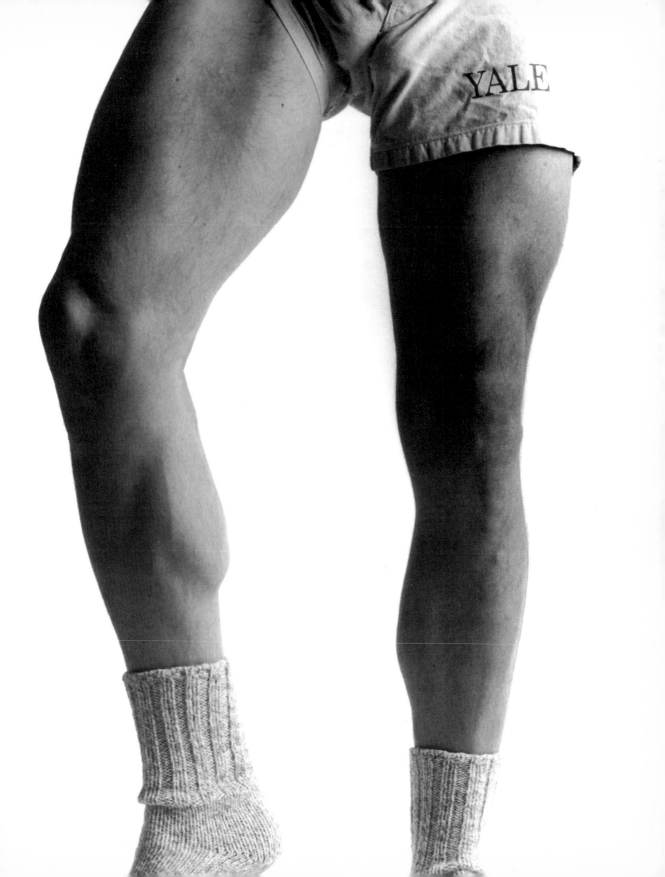

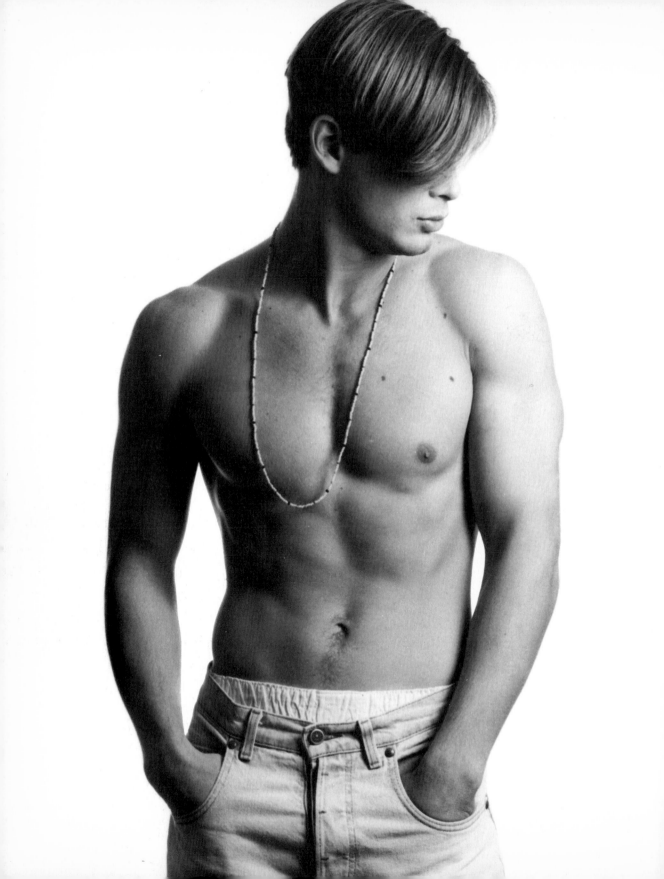

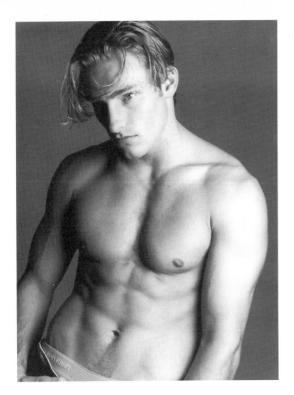
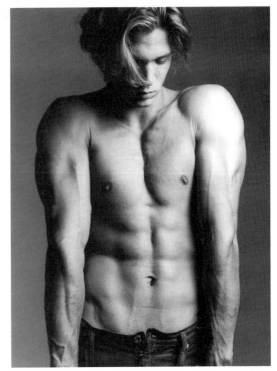
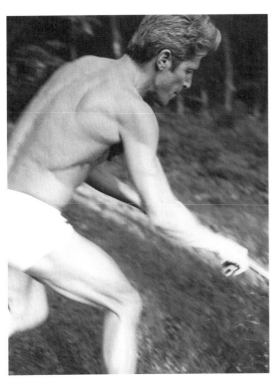
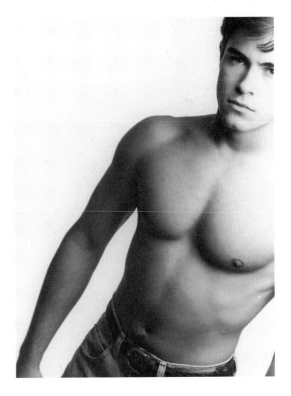

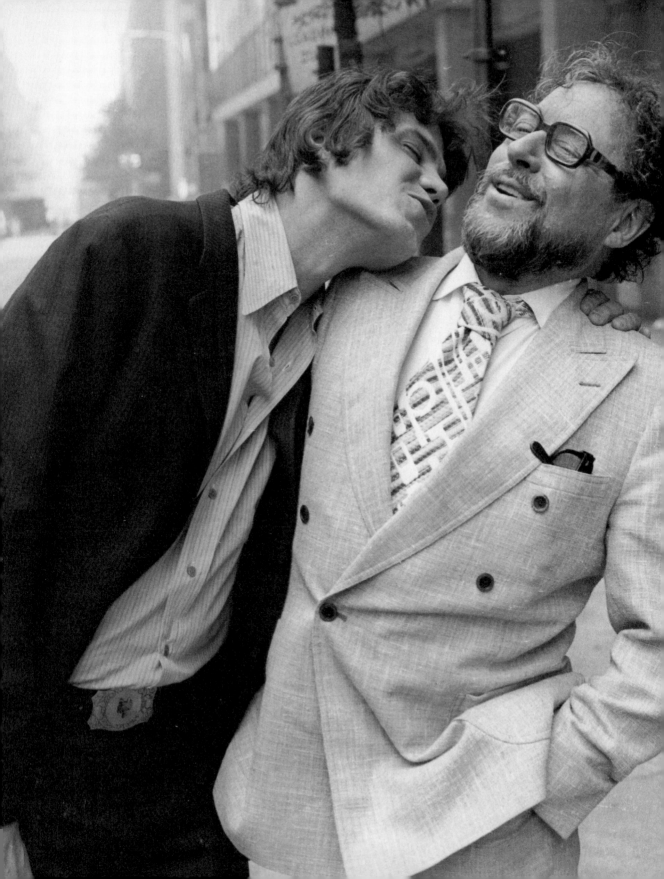

happy to take off their shirts and have their pictures taken, all you had to do was ask. And when you had a camera, you didn't have to worry about being a troll or a lech, you were an artist capturing a perfect moment.

Christopher doesn't take cabs everywhere the way Warhol did. He rides a bicycle from his Greenwich Village apartment to his TriBeCa studio. If he sees a beautiful boy he wants to photograph along the way, he'll just stop and ask.

When he was eating French toast at the Bagel Restaurant, the owner's son, Andrew, was his waiter.

"Are you an actor?" Christopher asked.

"Yeah, I'm an actor," said Andrew.

Andrew had taken some acting lessons, that's all. He's a student at New York University. He's nineteen, but Christopher still got permission from Andrew's parents before inviting him to the studio.

Christopher says he prefers shooting straight guys like Andrew than gay guys because they're usually less conscious of their looks. And he prefers men to women, because there's not as much effort involved in hunk photography. There are no hair, makeup, or wardrobe people here. All Andrew has to do is take off his shirt and do a few push-ups to pump up his pecs. Christopher's not interested in making people look a lot better than they really are, though his lighting favors abdominal muscles (plus the guys "crunch in" during the shoot for maximum abs).

OPPOSITE: *Tennessee Williams and friend by Christopher Makos*

BELOW: *Christopher Makos by Paul Washington*

Christopher's done with Andrew in less than a half hour, which is great because he's got a lot of portraits to do. Bergdorf-Goodman will hang them in their men's store.

Christopher tells Andrew and some other instant models that they're welcome to hang out. Bob Morris, a *New York Times* columnist, is coming and maybe they can all get mentions. Christopher's generous and democratic in a lot of ways. He's happy to share his

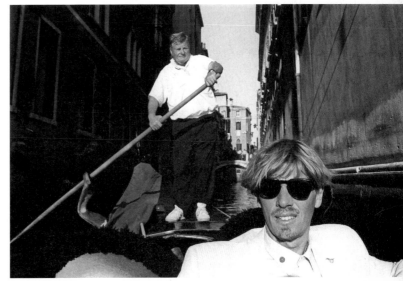

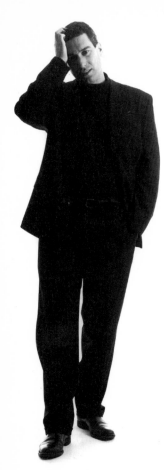

Bob Morris
by Christopher Makos

fame and gets so excited about his work that he says he'd show it in a laundromat, just as long as it gets out there.

Warhol said that he wished he could buy Christopher's energy, and it's hard to believe he's forty-six. Talking to Christopher is sometimes like trying to hold the attention of a pinball machine. He doesn't have time for books and usually doesn't read magazine articles unless he is mentioned.

What settles Christopher are his subjects. And to be in his studio you need beauty, wealth, or fame, or a hand in creating fame. Christopher learned a lot from Warhol. When he would check up on Christopher's nights out, Warhol always asked, "Did you meet somebody cute or famous?"

Not too long ago, I would have come to Christopher's studio as a writer, yet hoping he'd find me cute enough to photograph. But now that I know even plastic surgery can't make me beautiful, I've accepted my fate. I'm happy to sit in a corner here and watch these young people. And when I see how beautifully they photograph, I realize I wouldn't want to have my picture taken even if Christopher—for the hell of it—offered. I know I'll never be happy with what I saw. If I can't be a beauty, I'll try to be a worthy spectator.

Christopher's assistant reloads the camera while David Barton lounges on a couch, shirtless. He's maybe five-foot-four and his jeans shorts are so high up his muscle-bound legs that you can almost see his seminal vesicle. David's boyish face alone is cute enough to get him invited here, plus he's got a body that has already appeared in many of the muscleman publications.

Some join his Manhattan gym, the David Barton Gym, just to check him out or maybe feel his biceps if they can afford to hire him as a personal trainer. The motto of David's gym is "Look better with no clothes on."

"It's 'Look better naked,'" he corrects me.

David likes to wear as few articles of clothing as possible. There are photos of him in the Style section of the *Times* all the time. He'll be at a formal sit-down function wearing a tank top but still have diners in formal wear on either side of him, both looking happy with the seating arrangement.

"When I walk down the beach and every head turns, I feel damn good," he says. When he doesn't want to be noticed, he can always throw on a winter coat. Or wear a suit on the beach the way Nixon used to.

David's posing now with his wife, Susanne Bartsch. Susanne throws parties as an occupation. She's evidently very good at it, as she can afford a man named the Baroness to travel with her and zip her up. Foreign nightclubs fly Susanne and her entourage overseas and pay them large sums just to make an appearance. So Susanne, like David, is used to being ogled. Together, they never run out of poses. How do they get their teeth so white?

"Do you lose any romantic intimacy with all the attention you get?" I ask David.

"If I lose a few intimate moments, I accept that," he says.

David isn't surprised when I ask him to flex his biceps. He giggles when I touch it.

Up until now, I've been a happy voyeur on this trip, lucky just to watch. But now that I've copped a feel—even if it was only a photogenic biceps—I wonder if I've violated the purity of this trip. But then I look around Makos's stu-

David Barton
by Christopher Makos

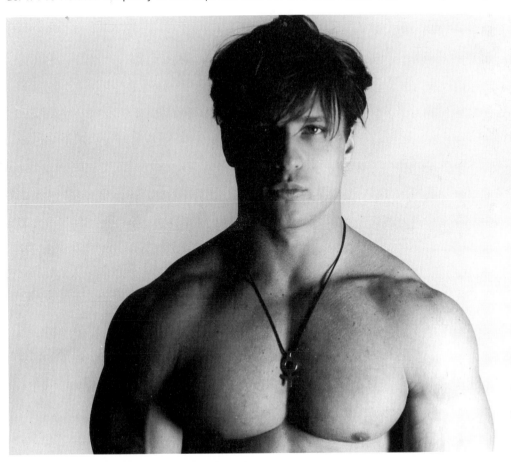

dio at all the framed portraits of bare torsos and remind myself that shirtless-hunk photographs—even the classic ones—can be used as a masturbatory aid. You're supposed to want to touch these guys, or touch yourself, when you see their photographs.

I've found this true of all the beautiful people I've met on this trip. I always felt some sexual curiosity. But when Makos boys come on to the camera, the feeling is a lot more immediate.

The shirtless hunk, though, means a lot more to me than something to whack off to. When I first saw the images by Makos and Weber and Warhol in *Interview,* I was a frustrated and miserable adolescent. Those photos were proof to me that beauty existed, something far beyond the lonely ugliness I was living through. I don't think I could ask more of beauty than that.

And now that the hunk has been accepted in prime time, ogled by suburban secretaries in Coke commercials, maybe pop culture is open to seeing other kinds of male beauty.

OPPOSITE: *Max by Josef Astor*

BELOW: *David Barton and Susanne Bartsch by Christopher Makos*

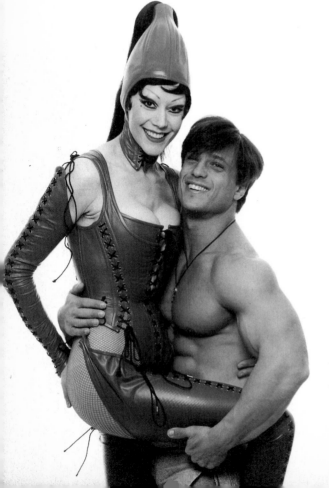

When I saw these photographs of Max, I didn't wonder whether his chest was hairy or smooth, or how big his biceps were. I just stared.

There is something deceivingly democratic about the hunk that this regal boy does not attempt to affect. By democratic I mean this: Guys who are inspired by the hunk image can go to the gym and attempt to look like him, or at least his arms and chest. (Of course, it's futile to attempt to become his twin, because his face is as flawless as his body.) But the beautiful boy does not offer a weight-lifting regimen you can follow. His beauty is his youth. It is effortless. You cannot aspire to his beauty, only feel privi-leged to admire it while he looks the other way. "He is in his own world," says his photographer Josef Astor. "It's not that he's thinking higher or lower thoughts, he's just some-where else." It is a dreamy beauty. In the past, he might have been an angel, or Tadzu in *Death in Venice.*

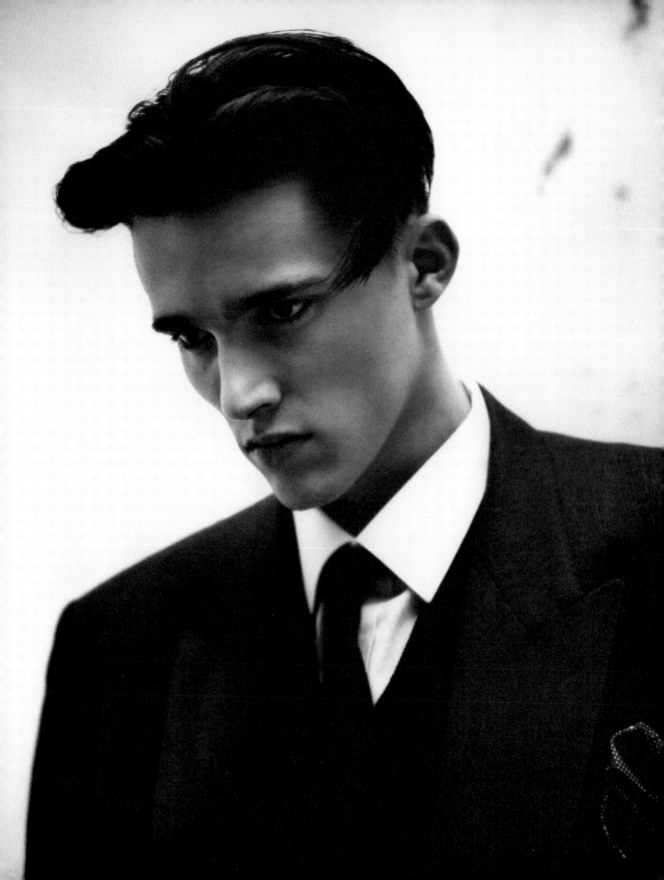

RIGHT: *Max*
by Josef Astor

OPPOSITE: *Botticelli*
in an Armani suit
by Josef Astor

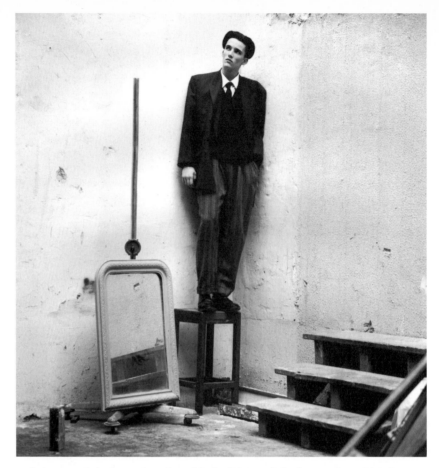

Astor says "aloofness is not cool today" (especially for men), and he does not expect his vision to wind up on billboards. But Astor's work is not hidden from sight, either. The amazing thing about the beauty trip today is that you don't have to be an indulged aristocrat, nor do you have to go underground to see your most wondrous vision of perfection.

Maybe your ideal image of beauty will not appear in *People* magazine's "50 Most Beautiful People" issue. But if you are willing to embrace beauty even as it eludes you, and have the patience to search for it everywhere except in your own mirror, you will see that fantasies are not illusions, that you can have photos of your dreams.

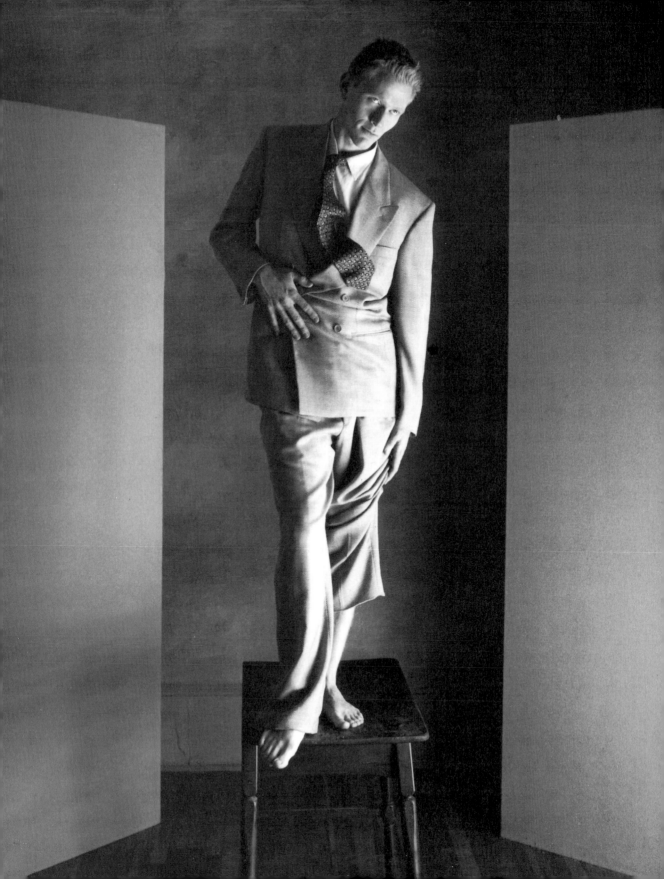

20

dorothy, Elly, and I get together and watch Lenda Murray win her fourth straight Ms. Olympia title.

Dorothy's working on a documentary about women bodybuilders now. Two months ago, Lenda's muscles scared her. Dorothy says she's not going to get her eyelashes dyed; she'd have to get them redyed every month and it's not worth the hassle. But she's going to start lifting weights in the new year.

Elly's not inspired by muscles, but says Lenda has "inner grace" to stay in Detroit and work with kids instead of moving to L.A. to try to become more famous. Elly says she calls goodness "inner grace" now instead of "beauty."

Elly's practical enough to admit that beauty exists and idealistic enough to want to make the pursuit of it as commonsensical and healthy as possible. "I'm interested only in things I can change," she says. "I can't change beauty, but maybe I can help change the way people try to achieve it.

Beauty, we all agree, is about an idealized moment that happens to a very few people during their youth. This doesn't mean beauty is only for teenagers. Not at all. I think of the enchantresses I met on this trip. Maria Snyder and Angeline are both in their mid-thirties, and Carmen is sixty-two. They cast a spell on strangers without trying. Their photos alone still allure me. But beautiful people exist, they are more beautiful than the rest of us, and they are most beautiful when they are young.

For years, whenever I tried to bring up the subject of beauty, friends would interrupt and say one of two things: "You don't look so bad, Ken," because they thought I was looking for a compliment, or "Real beauty, that comes from within," because they were putting me off.

I've come to understand why they were putting me off. To talk about beauty is to expose your own vanity, and once it's exposed, it's bound to be bruised.

But now that even Elly admits that physical beauty exists, I think about what she said at the beginning of this trip. Can "goodness," "inner beauty," "inner grace"—whatever you want to call it—"shine through" like she said? Is goodness visible?

I walk the streets of New York and stare at a lot of faces. I usually only give a second look to people I'd either want to kiss or photograph. But one day I walked down Broadway and tried to look for "inner beauty." I could tell a lot about people from just a quick glance—their likely political party affiliation, sexual preference, and taste in CDs. But though some faces looked friendlier than others, I couldn't see goodness. If we could spot goodness on sight, we'd all be spared a lot of bad relationships and smarmy elected officials.

But maybe I'm too secular and cynical a man, so I called Kenneth Woodward. I wanted to talk to him because he wrote a great book about how to become a saint, *Making Saints*. He's also the religion editor at *Newsweek*. In his thirty years of reporting on stigmatics, visionaries, healers, martyrs, and people who've devoted their lives to helping the poor, he says he's only twice encountered physical presences so commanding that he could actually feel a force (Billy Graham and Frank Sinatra), but he's never seen someone whose appearance signified their goodness. "Inner beauty" can be judged only by deeds and over time. It's futile, even dangerous, to think we can see virtue the same way we can spot beauty, or that inner beauty can always shine through.

It's also futile to think that beauty can guarantee love. As Carmen said, she never found her prince. With love, beauty really is in the eye of the beholder. Because love really does depend on more than just looks. At a crowded cocktail party, everybody is checking out the same couple of faces and bodies. Where we differ is who we'd meet at that party, who we'd want to hang out with, who we'd fall in love with, who we'd spend the rest of our lives with.

But even love doesn't diminish the yearning for beauty. Even though I'm in love, I haven't stopped wanting to be beautiful. I still think it is the simplest way to please people, like an offering. A beautiful face is easier to forgive, harder to say no to.

I'd hoped that with all the beautiful people I'd met on this trip, maybe one could give me the phone number of the plastic surgeon who could create perfect skin. But there are no secret numbers. All the best surgeons have been profiled in *People* or *Women's Wear Daily*. And the honest ones will tell you that beauty cannot be created. As remarkable as plastic surgery is—and it is the closest we've come to discovering the Fountain of Youth—at its best it can take maybe ten years off a face. It is not going to change my fate.

Dorothy is still awed by beauty but doesn't envy it as much as she used to. "I see how much of my personality developed because I wasn't a beauty," she says. "So when I talked to these beautiful people, it was hard to be envious when I realized I had so little in common with them. If I didn't ask them so many questions, there wouldn't have been much to say. And they weren't that interested in what I had to say. Now that I've faced beauty down, I don't think less of it. It would be great to be a beauty, but now I appreciate what I've got."

The reason this trip didn't turn ugly for me, either, is because I wasn't expecting anything from the beautiful people. If I'd been trying to get laid, or hoping to get invitations to their parties, I would have become bitter and resentful for being snubbed. To celebrate beauty is to create an elite. And inevitably when the elite get together, there are going to be a lot of rejections. Still, after I was able to look and look and look some more, and then finally be able to talk about beauty with other people instead of to myself, I was just grateful to know that this Alice in Wonderland world of beauty does exist. Hard as I tried, I'll never know what it's like to be beautiful. But I think that just having been able to go on this beauty trip may be as much a privilege as beauty itself.

Not long ago, I was looking at Bruce Weber's photos for the new Gianni Versace ad campaign with Sam Shahid, the man who art directs much of Weber's work.

"Youth and beauty," Sam said. "Ain't nothin' like it in the world."

I'd thought by then I'd be able to respond in one of two ways. Either: "I used to think so, but now that I've seen the beautiful people up close, their outer shells do nothing for me. Just last night, Kate Moss and Johnny Depp were having dinner at the table next to mine, and I didn't even glance over. I wouldn't have even known it was them if it hadn't been for the paparazzi."

Or: "You're right. There's nothing like youth and beauty. And by contemplating the finest portraits of the most beautiful people—in a controlled environment—I was led to a heavenly state."

But I was able to say neither. I will always stare at beauty. And my only glimpse of heaven has been what I've read in those near-death experience books.

Keats said that "Beauty is truth, truth beauty, – that is all / Ye know on earth, and all ye need to know." I am still trying to find out exactly what that means. I did find, however, that being truthful about beauty was the only way for me to realize that it is necessary for me to take another, entirely different trip. But before I do, I'm going to go get my teeth whitened.

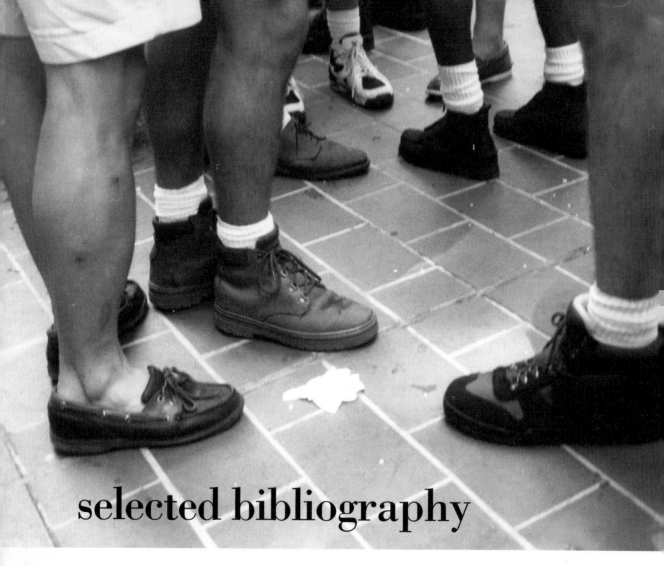

selected bibliography

Feet
by Christopher Makos

Angier, Natalie. "Fashion's Waif Look Makes Strong Women Weep," *The New York Times,* April 11, 1993.

Bachrach, Judy. "Eileen Ford," *People,* May 16, 1993.

Baldwin, James. *Giovanni's Room.* New York: The Dial Press, 1956.

Boadi, Michael and Guido. "Supermodel Super Weird?" *I-D,* June 1993.

Dell'Orefice, Carmen. *Staying Beautiful: Beauty Secrets and Attitudes from My Forty Years as a Model,* New York: Harper and Row, 1985.

Duka, John. "Weber's Naturalistic Eye on Men's Fashion," *The New York Times,* July 20, 1982.

"Eating Disorders," brochure published by the National Institute of Mental Health, U.S. Department of Health and Human Services, 1993.

Ford, Eileen. *Eileen Ford's Beauty Now and Forever.* New York: Simon and Schuster, 1977.

Hartocollis, Anemona. "What Price Beauty?" *New York Newsday,* June 28, 1992.

Johnson, Richard. "Star Shapers: Makeover MDs Eye Their Own Profiles," *Daily News,* February 2,1992.

Lynden, Patricia. "Behind the Scenes with a Dermatologist," *Allure,* July 1992.

Murphy, Mary. "Dolly Parton," *TV Guide,* November 27, 1993.

Plaskin, Glenn. "*Playboy* Interview: Calvin Klein," *Playboy,* May 1984.

Schonauer, David. "Eileen Ford on Money, Sex, and Power," *American Photo,* May–June 1993.

Spindler, Amy M. "Mixing Dada, Cher, Middle America," *The New York Times,* November 29, 1994

Weber, Bruce. *Hotel Room with a View.* Washington, D.C.: Smithsonian Institution Press, 1992.

Woodward, Kenneth. *Making Saints: How the Catholic Church Determines Who Becomes a Saint, Who Doesn't, and Why.* New York: Simon and Schuster, 1990.